VOLUME ONE HUNDRED AND THIRTY THREE

# ADVANCES IN CANCER RESEARCH

## Cancer Disparities

VOLUME ONE HUNDRED AND THIRTY THREE

# ADVANCES IN CANCER RESEARCH

## Cancer Disparities

Edited by

**MARVELLA E. FORD**
*Department of Public Health Sciences and Hollings Cancer Center, Medical University of South Carolina, Charleston, SC, United States*

**DENNIS K. WATSON**
*Department of Pathology and Laboratory Medicine and Hollings Cancer Center, Medical University of South Carolina, Charleston, SC, United States*

ELSEVIER

ACADEMIC PRESS
An imprint of Elsevier
elsevier.com

Academic Press is an imprint of Elsevier
50 Hampshire Street, 5th Floor, Cambridge, MA 02139, United States
525 B Street, Suite 1800, San Diego, CA 92101-4495, United States
The Boulevard, Langford Lane, Kidlington, Oxford OX5 1GB, United Kingdom
125 London Wall, London, EC2Y 5AS, United Kingdom

First edition 2017



ISBN: 978-0-12-809878-3
ISSN: 0065-230X

For information on all Academic Press publications
visit our website at https://www.elsevier.com/



*Publisher:* Zoe Kruze
*Acquisition Editor:* Zoe Kruze
*Editorial Project Manager:* Fenton Coulthurst
*Production Project Manager:* Surya Narayanan Jayachandran
*Senior Cover Designer:* Miles Hitchen

Typeset by SPi Global, India

# CONTENTS

# CONTRIBUTORS

**E.T. Brown**
Morehouse School of Medicine, Atlanta, GA, United States

**K. Cannady**
Hollings Cancer Center, Medical University of South Carolina, Charleston, SC, United States

**E. Cook**
University of Texas MD Anderson Cancer Center, Houston, TX, United States

**A. Evans-Knowell**
South Carolina State University, Orangeburg, SC, United States

**V.J. Findlay**
Hollings Cancer Center, Medical University of South Carolina, Charleston, SC, United States

**M.E. Ford**
Hollings Cancer Center, Medical University of South Carolina, Charleston, SC, United States

**T. Ginossar**
University of New Mexico, Albuquerque, NM, United States

**M. Gregoski**
Campbell University, Buies Creek, NC, United States

**C. Hoyo**
North Carolina State University, Raleigh, NC, United States

**C.H. Halbert**
Hollings Cancer Center, Medical University of South Carolina; Ralph H. Johnson Veterans Affairs Medical Center, Charleston, SC, United States

**K.D. Knight**
Hollings Cancer Center, Medical University of South Carolina, Charleston, SC, United States

**R. Kramer**
Medical University of South Carolina, Charleston, SC, United States

**A.C. LaRue**
Research Services, Ralph H. Johnson VAMC; Hollings Cancer Center, Medical University of South Carolina, Charleston, SC, United States

**R.L. Maguire**
North Carolina State University, Raleigh, NC, United States

**G. Magwood**
Medical University of South Carolina, Charleston, SC, United States

**S.K. Murphy**
Duke University Medical Center, Durham, NC, United States

**A. Napoles**
University of California, San Francisco, CA, United States

**L.L. Peterson**
Washington University School of Medicine, St. Louis, MO, United States

**L.J. Rice**
Hollings Cancer Center, Medical University of South Carolina, Charleston, SC, United States

**D.P. Turner**
Hollings Cancer Center, Medical University of South Carolina, Charleston, SC, United States

**A.C. Vidal**
Cedar-Sinai Medical Center, Los Angeles, CA, United States

# PREFACE

The National Cancer Institute defines cancer health disparities as:

> *Adverse differences in cancer incidence (new cases), cancer prevalence (all existing cases), cancer death (mortality), cancer survivorship, and burden of cancer or related health conditions that exist among specific population groups in the United States.*
>
> *https://www.cancer.gov/about-nci/organization/crchd/cancer-health-disparities-fact-sheet*

The contributors to cancer disparities are multifactorial. Therefore, a multidisciplinary research approach is required to identify these contributors and to develop solutions to addressing them.

The ultimate goal of cancer disparities research is to reduce risk and improve treatment and survivorship outcomes among members of groups that are disproportionately impacted by cancer. *Cancer Disparities*, the latest in the *Advances in Cancer Research* series, provides invaluable information on this exciting and fast-moving field of cancer research. This volume describes the complex interplay of contributors to cancer disparities, ranging from the micro- to macro-level, and based on the biological, social, and environmental determinants of health.

This latest volume presents the first of two issues on cancer disparities, and provides a broad introduction to a spectrum of factors contributing to these disparities. Topics range from basic biological pathways to social/behavioral and environmental factors influencing cancer disparities.

Chapter 1 by Dr. David P. Turner, "The Role of Advanced Glycation End-Products in Cancer Disparity," provides an overview of AGEs and AGE metabolites, their relationship to diet and metabolism, possible mechanisms of whereby AGE accumulation results in pathogenesis, including inflammation, and their contribution to cancer disparity. In addition, a discussion of future directions, including therapeutic targeting, is included.

In Chapter 2, "Disparities in Obesity, Physical Activity Rates, and Breast Cancer Survival," Dr. Marvella E. Ford and colleagues provide a concise summary of disparities in breast cancer mortality rates, and the relationship between weight, physical activity, and breast cancer mortality. The disparities in overweight/obesity and physical activity are discussed. Importantly, evidence-based breast cancer survivorship guidelines related to physical activity and weight management are provided. Taken together, the chapter provides a rational for a multilevel intervention approach to reduce obesity and cancer mortality.

Chapter 3 by Dr. Ashley Evans-Knowell and colleagues, "MicroRNAs and Their Impact on Breast Cancer, the Tumor Microenvironment, and Disparities," focuses on the current published literature that is involved in the study of microRNAs and their impact on breast cancer disparities. The chapter includes a discussion of microRNAs, circulating microRNAs, and their roles in cancer, including the microenvironment, and cancer disparities, as well as representing a unique therapeutic target. The information presented in the chapter significantly extends the discussion of the potential role of microRNAs as contributors to breast cancer disparities.

In Chapter 4, "Applying a Conceptual Framework to Maximize the Participation of Diverse Populations in Cancer Clinical Trials," Dr. Anna Napoles and colleagues show that despite their disproportionate burden of cancer, racial and ethnic minorities are less likely than others to participate in cancer clinical trials. The authors describe a conceptual framework of factors that can affect the degree of success in recruiting and retaining ethnically diverse populations in research, including awareness, opportunities, and acceptance barriers. Sociodemographic characteristics are additional moderators of participation in clinical trials. The authors apply the conceptual framework to three studies that included ethnically diverse populations across different population groups and contexts. This chapter thus provides a timely overview of causes of low recruitment and significantly, strategies that have worked well to facilitate recruitment of diverse populations into clinical trials.

Chapter 5, "Social Networks Across Common Cancer Types: The Evidence, Gaps, and Areas of Potential Impact," by Drs. LaShanta J. Rice and Chanita Hughes-Halbert examines the literature on social networks and cancer across the cancer continuum among adults. Despite findings of associations between social networks and survival, risk, and screening with cancer, none of the studies identified employed social networks as a mechanism for reducing health disparities, indicating that this may be an area for future intervention.

In Chapter 6, "Disparities in Cervical Cancer Incidence and Mortality: Can Epigenetics Contribute to Eliminating Disparities?" Dr. Rachel L. Maguire and colleagues provide an overview of disparities in cervical cancer incidence and mortality, disparities in cervical intraepithelial neoplasia incidence, human papillomavirus (HPV), cofactors of HPV infection and cervical intraepithelial neoplasia (CIN) progression, HPV genetics and epigenetics, and ethnic disparities and host epigenetics. As HPV infection and cofactor patterns do not vary considerably by race/ethnicity to explain disparities in cervical cancer incidence and mortality, the authors argue that increased attention to epigenetic mechanisms is warranted. This is based upon the observation that changes in epigenetic patterns occur as a result of HPV infection and subsequent CIN and cancer. Thus, the authors provide a discussion of host DNA methylation and assess the extent to which it may be incorporated into screening platforms to decrease cervical cancer incidence and mortality.

In summary, the chapters in this volume provide an important foundation for future cancer disparities research. The information presented highlights the fact that we have much to learn regarding the causes of, and solutions to, cancer disparities. Exciting opportunities exist to expand the evolving paradigm of cancer disparities research.

Marvella E. Ford
Dennis K. Watson

# ABOUT THE EDITORS

**Dr. Marvella E. Ford** is a tenured professor in the Department of Public Health Sciences at the Medical University of South Carolina (MUSC), where she is the associate director of Cancer Disparities at the National Institutes of Health/National Cancer Institute (NIH/NCI)-designated Hollings Cancer Center. She completed her undergraduate training at Cornell University and she completed her graduate and postdoctoral fellowship training at the University of Michigan.

Dr. Ford has led several federally funded cancer disparities-focused research grants, including an NIH/NCI P20 grant, in collaboration with Dr. Judith Salley from South Carolina State University, titled South Carolina Cancer Disparities Research Center (SC CaDRe). The goal of the SC CaDRe was to expand cancer disparities research in South Carolina while cultivating a diverse network of cancer researchers. The grant provided funding for cancer disparities research and supported cancer research training for underrepresented students and junior faculty in cancer research methods.

Additionally, Dr. Ford has collaborated as a multiple principal investigator, with Dr. Chanita Hughes-Halbert and Dr. Carolyn Britten, on an NIH/NCI-funded Minority-Based Community Oncology Research Program to increase the participation of diverse participants in cancer research. Dr. Ford has also served as a multiple principal investigator, with Dr. Nestor Esnaola, of an NIH/National Institute on Minority Health and Health Disparities grant titled "Improving Resection Rates among African Americans with NSCLC." The purpose of the study was to evaluate a strategy to improve the rates of receipt of surgery among African Americans with early-stage lung cancer.

Dr. Ford has also led several federally funded cancer research training programs in collaboration with three historically black colleges/universities (HBCUs) in South Carolina: Claflin University, South Carolina State University, and Voorhees College, as well as the University of South Carolina. The programs have been funded by the NIH/NCI and by the Department of Defense.

Dr. Ford is the author/coauthor of more than 85 published scientific papers, several of which include undergraduates from HBCUs as coauthors. She has also published nine book chapters.

**Dr. Dennis K. Watson** has a long-standing interest and expertise in the areas of cellular and molecular biology, gene discovery, cellular differentiation, and molecular oncology. During the initial stages of oncogene discovery, he was among the first to molecularly characterize the viral and cellular myc genes. He was also among the discoverers of the Ets gene family and has been directly responsible for the isolation and characterization of Ets gene products and their role in cellular proliferation, differentiation, and etiology of cancer. In addition to continuing to evaluate the role of specific Ets genes in cellular transformation, his laboratory has identified and functionally characterized genes with altered expression during cancer progression. His research program has expertise in using in vitro and in vivo loss-of-function and gain-of-function approaches and molecular analyses to examine the functional significance of altered expression and the regulatory networks that such changes control. Recent studies in Dr. Watson's laboratory have explored the role of regulatory circuitry in tumor cell interaction with the microenvironment.

Dr. Watson has an extensive track record in educating and providing mentorship to over 25 predoctoral students, 25 postdoctoral trainees, and 12 junior faculty. He has also been a member of the thesis committees for 56 other graduate students and is the leader of the MUSC College of Graduate Studies' Cancer Biology curriculum for predoctoral students. After more than a decade as research program leader for the MUSC-HCC Cancer Genes and Molecular Regulation Program, he was appointed the inaugural Associate Director for Education and Training in 2013. In this role, he chairs the career development committee of the MUSC-HCC K12 program and works with MUSC-HCC leadership to develop education and training initiatives.

CHAPTER ONE

# The Role of Advanced Glycation End-Products in Cancer Disparity

**D.P. Turner**[1]
Hollings Cancer Center, Medical University of South Carolina, Charleston, SC, United States
[1]Corresponding author: e-mail addresses: turnerda@musc.edu; Andrei.Budanov@vcuhealth.org

## Contents



## Abstract

While the socioeconomic and environmental factors associated with cancer disparity have been well documented, the contribution of biological factors is an emerging field of research. Established disparity factors such as low income, poor diet, drinking alcohol, smoking, and a sedentary lifestyle may have molecular effects on the inherent biological makeup of the tumor itself, possibly altering cell signaling events and gene expression profiles to profoundly alter tumor development and progression. Our understanding of

*Advances in Cancer Research*, Volume 133
ISSN 0065-230X
http://dx.doi.org/10.1016/bs.acr.2016.08.001

the molecular and biological consequences of poor lifestyle is lacking, but such information may significantly change how we approach goals to reduce cancer incidence and mortality rates within minority populations. In this review, we will summarize the biological, socioeconomic, and environmental associations between a group of reactive metabolites known as advanced glycation end-products (AGEs) and cancer health disparity. Due to their links with lifestyle and the activation of disease-associated pathways, AGEs may represent both a biological consequence and a bio-behavioral indicator of poor lifestyle which may be targeted within specific populations to reduce disparities in cancer incidence and mortality.

## 1. INTRODUCTION

Specific populations in the United States and across the world suffer disproportionately high levels of cancer incidence and mortality. Poor diet, low income, and sedentary lifestyle are interrelated socioeconomic and environmental factors that are known to contribute to cancer disparity. Significantly, these factors are most prevalent in African-American (AA) communities which often have the highest levels of cancer incidence and mortality. While socioeconomic and environmental factors are established contributors to cancer health disparity, it is becoming increasingly apparent that molecular differences in tumor biology may also play a significant role. The role of biological factors remains one of the most understudied areas of cancer disparity research. Evidence supporting inherent biological differences in race-specific tumors includes faster disease progression in AA men with prostate cancer, higher prevalence of triple negative breast cancer in AA women, and race-specific differences in the expression patterns of multiple key cancer-associated genes. Intriguingly, lifestyle choices may also have profound effects on tumor biology which may contribute to cancer disparity outcomes such as its earlier development and its progression to more aggressive disease. The molecular composition of the primary tumor plays a critical role in determining a life-threatening phenotype, and it is now apparent that the established socioeconomic and environmental risk factors that drive cancer disparity can have profound effects on tumor biology. Factors such as a poor diet and a lack of exercise can alter tumor-associated gene expression, noncoding RNAs, chromosomal abnormalities, and gene polymorphisms to contribute to health disparity outcomes (Kinseth et al., 2014; Powell & Bollig-Fischer, 2013; Reams et al., 2009). Our understanding of the molecular consequences of poor lifestyle on tumor biology and its contribution to cancer disparity is still in its infancy and is subject to substantial debate. However, approaches that define the biological consequences of cancer health disparity may not only increase our understanding of cancer etiology but also define novel therapeutic targets and potential biomarkers with which to reduce cancer incidence and mortality.

## 2. ADVANCED GLYCATION END-PRODUCTS

A group of lifestyle-linked reactive metabolites have recently come to the fore as a potential biological mechanism driving cancer disparity. Advanced glycation end-products (AGEs) are reactive metabolites produced by the nonenzymatic glycosylation of sugars to biological macromolecules such as protein, DNA, and lipids, in a process known as glycation (Fig. 1). Glycation is a complex and multistep process involving a series of condensation, rearrangement, fragmentation, and oxidation reactions driven by the Maillard reaction. Carbohydrates such as fructose and glucose are metabolized by specific molecular pathways to produce essential metabolites

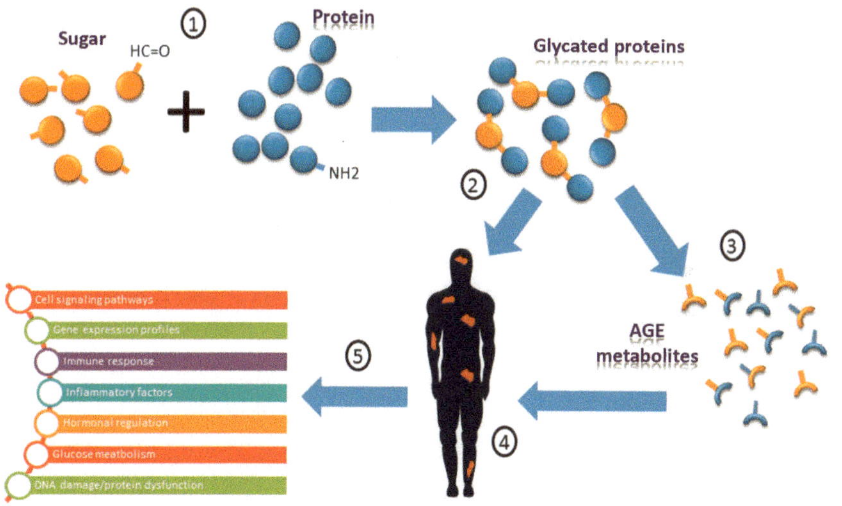


**Fig. 1** Through a series of condensation, rearrangement, fragmentation, and oxidation reactions driven by the Maillard reaction, sugars covalently attach to biological macromolecules such as proteins to form glycated adducts (1). Glycated proteins either accumulate in our tissues and organs (2) or are proteolytically degraded into reactive metabolites known as advanced glycation end-products or AGEs for short (3). AGEs can either further accumulate in our tissues and organs (4) or function as ligand to a number of receptor molecules. AGE accumulation can alter multiple biological pathways associated with multiple, if not all, chronic diseases (5).

that are required for metabolism and energy production (Uribarri et al., 2005, 2010). These essential metabolites produce carbohydrate intermediates which react with free amino groups to generate reactive carbonyl species (RCSs). These RCSs are AGE precursors which in turn non-enzymatically react with macromolecules such as proteins, lipids, and DNA to produce AGEs (Ansari & Raseed, 2008; Thornalley, 2003a, 2003b, 2008; Uribarri et al., 2005, 2010). Alternatively, RCSs can undergo further oxidation, dehydration, polymerization, and oxidative breakdown reactions to give rise to numerous other AGE metabolites. Clearance of AGEs is inefficient and they accumulate in our tissues and organs as we grow older with pathogenic effects (Fig. 1). Elevated AGE levels lead to protein dysfunction, protein cross-linking, decreased genetic fidelity, and aberrant cell signaling which can lead to increased activation of stress response pathways (Duran-Jimenez et al., 2009; Guimaraes, Empsen, Geerts, & van Grunsven, 2010; Riehl, Nemeth, Angel, & Hess, 2009). AGEs contribute to the development and complications associated with most chronic diseases including diabetes, cardiovascular disease, arthritis, and neurodegenerative disorders to name a few (Ansari & Rasheed, 2010; Singh, Barden, Mori, & Beilin, 2001). Further, disease states such as dyslipidemia, hypertension, and hyperglycemia are critical components of multiple diseases that play a fundamental role in increasing AGE accumulation. Significantly, all of these chronic disease states demonstrate significant health disparity, particularly among AAs.

## 3. AGE METABOLITES, LIFESTYLE, AND HEALTH DISPARITY

Apart from their endogenous buildup during glucose metabolism, AGEs are also accumulated as a consequence of lifestyle. The total levels of AGEs are a result of: (1) endogenous production during processes such as glucose metabolism, (2) exogenous intake and accumulation from diet and poor lifestyle factors, and (3) excretion from the body in urine and feces (Fig. 2). It is estimated that around 10–30% of exogenous AGEs are absorbed in the gut but only a third of those are excreted in urine and feces (Cho, Roman, Yeboah, & Konishi, 2007; Uribarri et al., 2010). Over the last few decades, the hallmarks of the Western lifestyle—an unhealthy diet combined with a sedentary lifestyle—have increased sharply. This has led to an increase in the contribution of exogenous sources of AGE accumulation,

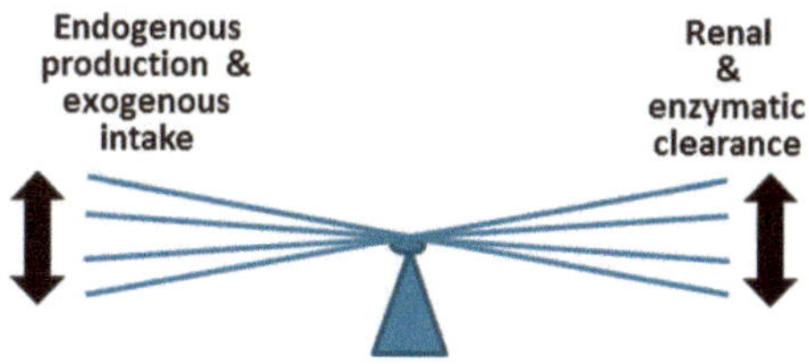


**Fig. 2** AGE accumulation is a balance between their endogenous and exogenous production and their excretion and enzymatic clearance from the body.

resulting in earlier aging, earlier disease onset, and worsening disease complications.

## 3.1 Diet

Many foods are significant contributors to exogenous AGE accumulation (Uribarri et al., 2007, 2005, 2010; Vlassara, 2005). The typical Western diet, which is high in sugar, protein, and fat, and low in fruits, grains, and vegetables, is particularly AGE laden and associated with increased chronic disease risk (Uribarri et al., 2007, 2005, 2010; Vlassara, 2005). The way that foods are cooked also has a significant effect on total AGE content. AGEs are naturally present in uncooked meats. Frying, grilling, or roasting (i.e., dry heat) accelerates the formation of AGEs in food by approximately 10-fold. Similarly, food processing and manufacturing also accelerate AGE formation and are now a major source of exogenous AGEs. Food manufacturers add AGEs directly to foods in order to improve their appearance and taste. Significantly, processed foods now represent one of the most common food items found in grocery shopping carts especially in low-income families who live in areas with few healthy food choices.

## 3.2 Obesity

Hyperglycemia, hyperlipidemia, and elevated oxidative stress are common features of obesity that increase the endogenous AGE accumulation pool. Decreases in AGEs correlate with reduced body weight and body fat content (Yoshikawa, Miyazaki, & Fujimoto, 2009). The AGE metabolite CML is extensively studied in animal models of disease, especially within the context of food content and is often used as an indicator of AGE levels in biological systems (Ames, 2008; Han et al., 2013). The differentiation of human preadipocytes to adipocytes (fat accumulation) is associated with increased CML levels and may have significant effects on adipose tissue and adipocyte regulation. CML accumulation in the fatty livers of obese individuals is associated with increased steatosis. Increased levels of the AGE precursor methylglyoxyl (MG) are also associated with obesity. Studies in obese rats have shown MG accumulation in serum and fat tissue. AGEs may play an important role in aberrant adipose tissue regulation by altering the expression and secretion of inflammatory adipokines to alter cell signaling pathways and gene expression profiles.

## 3.3 Sedentary Lifestyle

Recent data from the European Prospective Investigation into Cancer and Nutrition Study concludes that a sedentary lifestyle poses twice the risk of premature death as being overweight or obese (Ekelund et al., 2015). As shown in human (Yoshikawa et al., 2009) and animal studies (Boor et al., 2009) a more active lifestyle can help maintain a stable level or even reduce circulatory AGE accumulation. In obese rats, regular moderate exercise reduced advanced glycation early diabetic nephropathy, lowered plasma AGE-associated fluorescence as well as overall renal AGE content (Boor et al., 2009). Exercise training of late middle-aged rats lowered AGE accumulation and attenuated cardiac fibrosis and collagen cross-linking resulting in a reduction in age-related mortality between late middle age and senescence (Wright, Thomas, Betik, Belke, & Hepple, 2014). In a type 2 diabetes rat model, regular moderate exercise protocol is more effective in reducing serum level of AGEs than an irregular, severe exercise program (Salama, 2013). In nondiabetic middle-aged women, a 12-week lifestyle modification consisting of an initial educational session followed by encouragement showed that the number of daily walking steps significantly correlated with lower AGE levels. Reduced body weight, body fat, and serum HDL-cholesterol levels are associated with decreased AGE (Yoshikawa et al., 2009). In patients with hypertension, physical activity inhibited the progression of left ventricular hypertrophy via a reduction in AGE levels (Akihiro, 2014).

## 3.4 Behavioral Risk Factors

Behavioral risk factors such as tobacco use and alcohol consumption are also associated with elevated exogenous AGE levels. AGE levels are significantly higher in chronic alcohol drinkers (Kalousová, 2004) and acetaldehyde-derived AGEs promote alcoholic liver disease (Hayashi, 2013). AGE precursors are present in tobacco extracts and tobacco smoke and can rapidly react with biological macromolecules to form AGE metabolites. Tissue accumulation of AGEs is higher in smokers than in nonsmokers and tobacco-derived AGEs have been demonstrated to accumulate on vessel walls and in the eye (Cerami et al., 1997; Nicholl & Bucala, 1998). Both smoking and alcohol intake as well as lack of sleep were positively correlated with increased AGEs in the skin of Japanese men and women (Nomoto, Yagi, Arita, Ogura, & Yonei, 2012).

## 3.5 Significance to Ethnic and Racial Health Disparity

Environmental, socioeconomic, and behavioral risk factors including low income, poor diet, lack of exercise, excessive drinking, and smoking are prevalent in AA communities and are responsible for increased AGE accumulation (Fig. 3). At over 27%, poverty rates within AAs are among the highest in the country (http://www.stateofworkingamerica.org). Low-income status is associated with the utilization of cheap, unhealthy, and highly processed foods which are AGE laden and promote obesity. Food deserts are areas with poor or no availability of fresh fruits, vegetables, and other healthful whole foods (i.e., foods with low AGE content). This is largely due to a lack of grocery stores, farmers' markets, and healthy food providers. Food deserts are largely found in impoverished areas and AAs are statistically more likely to live in designated food deserts than other populations. Additionally, AAs are 1.5 times as likely to be obese as non-Hispanic Whites. AA women and girls are 80% more likely to be obese than their

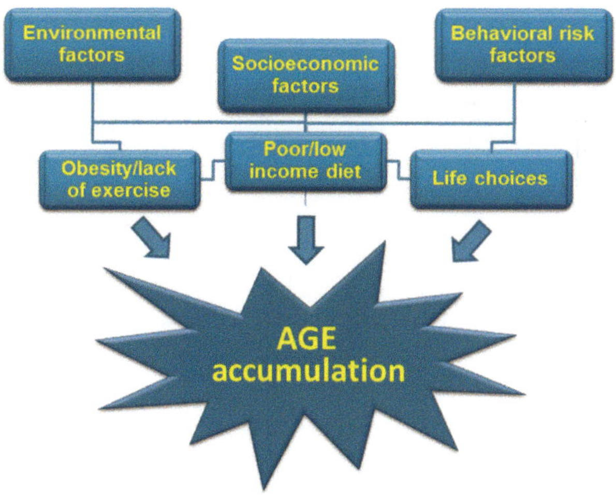


**Fig. 3** Environmental, socioeconomic, and behavioral risk factors including low income, poor diet, lack of exercise, excessive drinking, and smoking are lifestyle disparity factors that are particularly prevalent in our AA communities which are also responsible for increased AGE accumulation.

non-Hispanic white counterparts (http://minorityhealth.hhs.gov/). A higher percentage of AAs report getting little of no exercise and do not meet federal physical activity guidelines. It is estimated that only 50% of AA men and 35% of AA women do not meet Federal Aerobic Physical Activity Guidelines (https://www.heart.org). Due to the common links between these factors that drive health disparity and the increased accumulation of AGEs, elevated AGE levels may influence risk of cancer and define a metabolic susceptibility difference driving cancer and cancer health disparity.

## 4. MECHANISMS OF AGE PATHOGENICITY

Endogenous and exogenous AGE accumulation can have multiple pathogenic consequences to the function of biological macromolecules. AGEs accumulate in both the intracellular and extracellular compartments to contribute to the onset of multiple diseases, as well as subsequent disease complications. Elevation of the AGE accumulation pool is associated with increases in protein dysfunction, aberrant activation of cellular signaling cascades, and compromised genetic integrity. It is not known if the same AGE-mediated pathogenic effects identified in other diseases function in the tumor microenvironment or to what extent AGEs derived as a consequence of health disparity contribute to tumor growth.

### 4.1 Protein Dysfunction

The formation and accumulation of AGEs can alter protein function via a number of interrelated mechanisms including protein–protein cross-linking, charge distribution changes, decreased protein half-life, compromised structural integrity, and altered protein conformation. AGE effect on a specific protein depends upon several factors including the inherent reactivity of specific amino groups, glucose concentration, and protein half-life (Wautier & Schmidt, 2004). The nonenzymatic glycosylation of proteins results in the formation of protein cross-links on long-lived proteins such as collagen and elastin. AGE cross-link formation accumulates over time and is accelerated when glucose levels are high, as seen in diabetic patients. AGE cross-links have been shown to form at multiple sites within the collagen molecule resulting in increased protein half-life and a stiffening of tissues and arterial walls. This may contribute to cardiovascular complications such as atherosclerosis. AGE cross-linking also results in the aggregation of lens crystallins causing lens opacification and diabetic retinopathy (Ahmed, 2005). The glycation of laminin and fibronectin in diabetic rats decreases the key processes of neuronal migration and differentiation which can be prevented by treatment with the AGE inhibitor aminoguanidine (Duran-Jimenez et al., 2009).

## 4.2 Aberrant Cell Signaling

AGEs are associated with significant and interrelated increases in the aberrant activation of cell signaling cascades. AGEs function as ligand activators for a number of transmembrane receptors. The best studied is the receptor for advanced glycation end-products (RAGEs). RAGE (or AGER) is a member of the immunoglobulin superfamily and is highly expressed during embryonic development. Normal physiological functions of RAGE focus on immune response regulation and include embryonic neuronal growth, myogenesis, dendritic cell mobilization, T cell regulation, stem cell migration, and osteoclast maturation. Levels of RAGEs are relatively low in adult tissues and its upregulation is observed in multiple chronic diseases associated with health disparity including cancer. The main mechanistic consequence of RAGE activation by AGE is the increased activation of stress response pathways which also represent potential biological mechanisms of cancer health disparity.

### *4.2.1 Immune-Mediated Inflammation*

Recent research indicates that the biological immune response is implicated in cancer health disparity (Kinseth et al., 2014; Martin, Starks, & Ambs, 2013; Rose et al., 2010). An examination of expression differences based upon tumor composition shows that cytokine signaling associated with an increased immune response is the predominant pathway increased in AA prostate cancer patients (Kinseth et al., 2014). Upon closer analysis, the majority of race-specific differential gene expression was found in the stromal compartment of the tumor (Kinseth et al., 2014). A similar race-specific increase in immune response gene copy number and gene expression was seen in matched radical prostatectomy tissues (Rose et al., 2010) and in Gleason 6 prostate tumors (Reams et al., 2009). In breast cancer, AA race is a significant risk factor for elevated cytokine levels after controlling for other known risk factors (Park & Kang, 2013).

RAGE is expressed on the surface of most immune cells types and is functionally linked to an increased recruitment of immune cells in a wide range of diseases (Riehl et al., 2009; Rojas et al., 2011). Its stimulation by ligands such as AGE induces the transcriptional activation immune master regulators such as NFkB, STAT3, and HIF1α. This results in the increased expression and secretion of regulatory cytokines such as IL1, IL6, and TNFα (Riehl et al., 2009; Rojas et al., 2011) to produce a persistent and cyclic increase in immune-mediated inflammation. Loss of RAGE in inflammatory mouse models confers resistance to induced skin carcinogenesis (Riehl et al., 2009; Rojas et al., 2011). In castrate-sensitive and castrate-resistant prostate cancer cell lines, AGE is identified as the ligand for RAGE interactions, but other ligands (S100B or amphoterin) are not (Allmen, Koch, Fritz, & Legler, 2008).

### 4.2.2 Oxidative Stress

Clinical and epidemiological evidence identifies AA race as an independent risk factor for elevated oxidative stress and increased reactive oxygen species (ROS) (Fisher et al., 2012; Morris et al., 2012). Nicotinamide adenine dinucleotide phosphate (NAPDH) oxidase catalyzes the reduction of superoxide radicals to generate ROS. Significantly, AA human umbilical vein endothelial cells show higher levels of nitric oxide, lower superoxide dismutase activity, and increased expression of the NAPDH oxidase subunit p47phox protein than their Caucasian counterparts (Feairheller et al., 2011). ROS derived from NAPDH oxidases may elevate the risk of cancer, and targeting NAPDH oxidases can inhibit tumor growth (Weyemi, Redon, Parekh, Dupuy, & Bonner, 2013). ROS-generating NADPH oxidases are a critical mediator in oncogenic H-Ras-induced DNA damage (Weyemi et al., 2013). Poor diet, reduced physical activity, alcohol consumption, and cigarette smoking not only increase the AGE accumulation levels but also significantly increase the oxidative stress levels in our body (Aseervatham, Sivasudha, Jeyadevi, & Arul Ananth, 2013; Dato et al., 2013), but it is not known if the two are linked.

In multiple chronic diseases, there is a well-established mechanistic link between AGE and elevated oxidative stress (Bansal et al., 2012; Guimaraes et al., 2010; Morita, Yano, Yamaguchi, & Sugimoto, 2013; Peppa, Uribarri, & Vlassara, 2008; Stirban et al., 2008, 2006; Wautier et al., 2001). This may also result in a persistent and cyclic increase in ROS levels in tumor cells. Another critical pathogenic consequence of the AGE–RAGE pathway is an increase in reactive oxygen intermediates (ROIs) and the generation of ROS both in vitro and in vivo (Bansal et al., 2012; Guimaraes et al., 2010; Morita et al., 2013; Peppa et al., 2008; Stirban et al., 2008, 2006; Wautier et al., 2001). This can lead to aberrant activation of cell signaling cascades and altered gene expression and function as well as DNA damage (Bansal et al., 2012; Guimaraes et al., 2010; Morita et al., 2013; Peppa et al., 2008; Stirban et al., 2008, 2006; Wautier et al., 2001). Reactive intermediates generated during AGE formation (i.e., Schiff's bases and Amadori products) can directly increase ROS production to further promote stress responses (Li, Sigmon, Babcock, & Ren, 2007; Rojas, Mercadal, Figueroa, & Morales, 2008; Sparvero et al., 2009). In a potential feed-back loop, oxidizing conditions and ROS presence can further promote the formation of AGEs via the formation of AGE precursors such as MG (Baynes, 2001; Chang & Wu, 2006; Desai et al., 2010; Yao & Brownlee, 2010). Consuming foods that increase AGE levels in the body such as red meat, and those with high fat and carbohydrate content increases oxidative stress and ROS levels. Significantly, antioxidants can inhibit AGE induced changes in glucose consumption and lower ROS levels (de Arriba et al., 2003). Furthermore, multiple studies in other diseases indicate that the AGE–RAGE signaling axis induces NAPDH oxidase activity and elevated ROS levels. Pharmacological inhibition of NAPDH oxidases inhibits AGE-mediated generation of ROIs and AGE-stimulated effects are suppressed in gp91phox-null macrophages (Wautier et al., 2001).

## 4.3 DNA Damage

ROS and AGEs represent some of the most reactive metabolites generated during human metabolism and both have an increased propensity for increasing levels of genotoxic insult to reduce genetic integrity. The biological significance of oxidative DNA damage to cancer has been well established, but its etiology is still not fully understood. The perpetual feed-forward loop observed between AGE and ROS leading to a cyclic increase in oxidative stress levels may have critical consequences to cancer-associated DNA damage, but the oxidative-dependent and -independent implications of AGE-mediated DNA damage have not yet been assessed. Significantly, AGE-DNA adducts in noncancer cell lines produce multibase deletions, base-pair substitutions, tandem mutations, and base-pair additions/deletions (Barea & Bonatto, 2008). DNA nucleotides readily react with RCSs to form several species of dNTP-AGE which are potentially genotoxic and mutagenic (Barea & Bonatto, 2008; Wuenschell et al., 2010). The major nucleotide AGEs are 3-(2′-deoxyribosyl)-6,7-dihydro-6,7-dihydroxyimidazo[2,3-*b*] purin-9(8)one (dGG), N2-carboxymethyl-deoxyguanosine (CMdG), and 5-glycolyldeoxycytidine (gdC) derived from the metabolite glyoxal, and

3-(2′-deoxyribosyl)-6,7-dihydro-6,7-dihydroxy-6-methylimidazo-[2,3-*b*] purine-9(8)one (dG-MG) and N2-(1-carboxyethyl)-deoxyguanosine (CEdG) derived from the metabolite methylglyoxal. Carboxymethyl-2′deoxyadenosine (CMdA) was recently identified by HPLC and LC/MS spectroscopy from glycoxidative reactions of deoxyadenosine and reactive carbohydrates D-glucose, D-ribose, and L-ascorbic acid (Thornalley, 2003b). Hydrolysis of CMdA gives carboxymethyl adenine which is present in human and calf-thymus DNA samples (Thornalley, 2003b). The quantitative assessment of dNTP-AGE adducts and their molecular links with oxidative DNA damage are of likely pathogenic and diagnostic significance and may represent race-specific surrogate measures of metabolic control linked to poor lifestyle and cancer. Immunohistochemical (IHC) and immunofluorescent (IF) staining showed elevated AGE levels in prostate tumor tissue compared to noncancer prostate tissue.

## 5. AGEs, CANCER, AND CANCER DISPARITY

Many of the risk factors associated with cancer disparity such as poor diet, lack of exercise, and obesity are also associated with the increased accumulation of AGEs. However, while several studies have investigated the role of RAGE in carcinogenesis, investigations regarding the functional contribution of AGEs to the onset and growth of cancer and their potential role as a lifestyle-linked biological factor contributing to cancer disparity are lacking. AGE presence in human tumors was first demonstrated in larynx, breast, and colon by IHC staining (van Heijst, Niessen, Hoekman, & Schalkwijk, 2005) and has since been shown to be also elevated in prostate tumors (Foster et al., 2014).

### 5.1 Prostate Cancer

Exogenous AGE treatment of immortalized prostate cancer cells promotes cell growth, migration, and invasion (Rodriguez-Teja et al., 2014). In prostate tumors, AGE-modified basement membrane in the form of collagen cross-linking promotes the invasive properties of prostate epithelial cells and correlates with decreased survival (Rodriguez-Teja et al., 2014). Circulating levels of the AGE metabolite carboxymethyl-lysine are significantly higher in serum from high-grade prostate cancer patients (Gleason grades 7–10) compared to that observed in low grade (Gleason grades 4–6) (Foster et al., 2014; Turner, 2015). Significantly, when stratified by race, circulating and tumoral AGE levels were significantly higher in serum and tissue from AA prostate cancer patients compared to Caucasian (Foster et al., 2014; Turner, 2015). This was observed in low-grade and high-grade tumors. Furthermore, like AGE, highest levels of RAGEs were observed in the tumor tissue compared to noncancer tissue with highest levels again being observed in AA samples (Foster et al., 2014; Turner, 2015). RAGE itself is overexpressed in a variety of tumor types (Riehl et al., 2009). Studies support a direct link between RAGE activation and proliferation, survival, migration, and invasion of tumor cells (Riehl et al., 2009; Rojas et al., 2011). Blockade of RAGE suppresses tumor growth in two independent mouse models (Riehl et al., 2009; Rojas et al., 2011). Silencing of RAGE reduces prostate-specific antigen expression and inhibits cell proliferation in prostate cancer cell lines and tumor growth in Nude mice (Elangovan et al., 2012). Studies show that the V-domain of RAGEs preferentially interacts with AGEs on prostate cancer cells over other ligands (Allmen et al., 2008). Recently the AGE–RAGE signaling axis has been shown to promote prostate cancer cell proliferation by increasing retinoblastoma (Rb) phosphorylation and degradation (Bao et al., 2015). Compared to controls, patients with elevated levels of circulating AGEs associated with increased risk of prostate cancer (Yang et al., 2015).

## 5.2 Breast Cancer

As for prostate, AGE treatment increases the growth, migratory, and invasive properties of breast cancer cell lines (Sharaf et al., 2015). In MCF7 breast cancer cells, the diabetes drug metformin inhibits AGE-mediated stimulation of growth by suppressing RAGE expression (Ishibashi, Matsui, Takeuchi, & Yamagishi, 2013). In studies examining AGE content in tumors, mass spectrometry analysis identified several AGE-modified proteins with known functional significance to breast cancer (Korwar et al., 2012).

## 5.3 Pancreatic Cancer

The potential link between diet and cancer has been supported by studies in pancreatic cancer. When analyzing dietary consumption of AGEs and pancreatic cancer in the NIH-AARP diet and health study, dietary-derived AGEs were associated with a modest increase in risk of pancreatic cancer and may partially explain its positive association with red meat (Jiao et al., 2015). Cooked red meat is a significant source of exogenous AGE, and men who consumed the most red meat had the highest risk of pancreatic cancer. However, alternative studies have failed to provide support for an association between AGE levels and pancreatic cancer risk (Grote et al., 2012).

### 5.4 Other Cancers

In colon cancer, activation of the AGE–RAGE signaling axis through a high AGE diet increased colon cancer development in rats (Shimomoto et al., 2012). AGE strongly induced the proliferation of primary acute myeloid leukemia via aberrant MAPK, PI3K, and JAK/STAT signaling (Kim et al., 2008).

## 6. TARGETING AGE BIOLOGY

As previously discussed, AGE accumulation is a significant pathogenic consequence of both endogenous and exogenous factors that promote multiple disease phenotypes. Several AGE-targeting drugs have been developed for the treatment of diabetes and neurodegenerative disorders (Rahbar, 2007) but there use as a potential cancer therapeutic has yet to be examined. Additionally given the link between AGEs and the socioeconomic and the environmental factors that contribute to cancer disparity, opportunities also exist to target AGE levels in our bodies through changes in lifestyle.

### 6.1 Drug Targeting

Strategies to target AGE biology for therapeutic gain are centered on the prevention of AGE formation and the reversal of AGE cross-links. Direct AGE-targeting drugs fall into two categories, AGE inhibitors and AGE breakers. AGE inhibitors target the AGE precursors formed during the Maillard reaction. Such prevention agents include dietary antioxidants (benfotiamine, pyridoxamine, vitamin C, vitamin E) which prevent the formation of the free radicals to inhibit oxidative AGE precursor development. Natural products such as resveratrol and curcumin through their antioxidant and antiinflammatory properties have also shown the AGE-inhibiting potential. Aminoguanidine is a nucleophilic hydrazine compound that scavenges RCSs and forms adducts with AGE precursors including MG. Clinical trials have shown that aminoguanidine prevents nephropathy, peripheral neuropathy, and retinopathy but has significant toxicity issues. Pyridoxamine (vitamin B complex) is another AGE precursor scavenger, has shown a similar beneficial effect as aminoguanidine, and has less toxicity issues. Metformin is a guanidine compound successfully used in the treatment of type 2 diabetes for a number of years (Yamagishi et al., 2008). Metformin has also showed some promise in the treatment of cancer but remains controversial (Kasznicki, Sliwinska, & Drzewoski, 2014; Pulito et al., 2013; Suissa & Azoulay, 2014). Metformin has been shown to inhibit the formation of AGEs and prevents cardiovascular defects associated with increased glycation (Yamagishi et al., 2008). Due to their irreversible nature and effects on protein dysfunction, AGE breakers are an attractive option for targeting AGE accumulation levels. Alagebrium (ALT711) selectively cleaves glucose-associated AGE cross-links by breaking carbon–carbon bonds between carbonyl groups. In diabetic animal studies, treatment with this drug reduces stiffness in arteries, improves endothelial dysfunction, preserves pressure-induced vasodilation, and reverses heart defects through decreases in AGE and RAGE levels (Yamagishi et al., 2008). However, studies in humans have yet to show similar promise.

## 6.2 Lifestyle Change

Reducing AGE levels for therapeutic gain may also be achieved through lifestyle change. Reducing AGE accumulation through self-management strategies may represent a novel paradigm for monitoring symptom status and promoting health behavior modification through cancer prevention initiatives arising through health and nutritional education and community outreach. This would allow for intensive risk reduction and improved identification of high-risk patients requiring defined dietary and physical activity intervention aimed at reducing the rate of AGE accumulation to reduce disease symptoms. While the accumulation of AGEs in our tissues and organs cannot be prevented, we can make changes to our everyday lifestyle to keep their accumulation at a minimum. Avoiding foods associated with a Western diet (i.e., high in protein, sugar, and fat as well as the use of processed foods) can significantly affect the rate at which AGEs accumulate in our bodies. Cooking foods with moist heat (boiling, steaming) rather than dry heat (frying, grilling) or substituting high-sugar, oil-based marinades with lemon juice, vinegar, and tomato juice (acidic marinades) can also drastically reduce exogenous AGE intake from the foods we consume. Along with dietary changes, taking steps to change a sedentary lifestyle toward a more active will prevent further AGE accumulation.

## 7. CONCLUDING REMARKS

The concept suggesting that AGE metabolites represent a biological consequence of lifestyle contributing to cancer disparity is a novel approach to explaining the increased incidence and mortality observed within diverse populations and may identify novel avenues for therapeutic and lifestyle intervention. From the translational perspective, a greater understanding regarding the role of AGEs in cancer and cancer disparity may:

**(1)** Provide a greater biological understanding of the potential benefits of lifestyle changes and their contribution to cancer disparity. Given the potential benefits of lifestyle changes and the role of lifestyle-associated AGEs in promoting disease phenotypes (Turner, 2015), multi-disciplinary efforts may significantly impact cancer prevention initiatives arising through health and nutritional education and community outreach efforts.

**(2)** Establish a role for AGE-mediated increases in stress response and DNA damage as mechanisms contributing to cancer disparity and tumor progression. Due to the higher complications and deaths associated with cancer in specific populations, a greater understanding of the risk factors and biological links associated with cancer disparity will significantly impact minority health.

**(3)** Set the stage for developing metabolite-based, noninvasive possibly race-specific prognostic markers. The accumulation of AGE metabolites may represent a distinct common disease risk factor associated with early recognition of cancer growth and/or progression. This would allow for intensive risk reduction and improved identification of high-risk patients requiring defined treatment.

**(4)** Define novel pathways for therapeutic intervention that would significantly impact cancer health disparity. Drug-targeting AGE metabolites have been developed for the treatment of diabetes and neurodegenerative disorders (Yamagishi et al., 2008). Further innovative insights may support targeting AGEs as a dual treatment option and identify protective factors that may underlie cancer disparity.

Sparse information exists about the genetic and biological factors that contribute to differential cancer survival and mortality rates observed in race-specific backgrounds. Associating the mechanistic links between glycation and cancer biology has not been examined in detail within the context of a race-specific background. In order to increase our mechanistic understanding of race-specific differences in tumor biology, we need to develop innovative molecular models with which to test working hypothesis and future potential treatments. The use of primary prostate tumor and patient-derived xenograft models in particular may successfully demonstrate race-specific differences in biological pathways which may be molecularly or genetically manipulated in future studies.

## ACKNOWLEDGMENTS

D.P.T.'s work was supported in part by grants from the National Institute of Health/National Cancer Institute (CA176135-Turner, CA194469-Turner, and CA157071-Ford).

## REFERENCES

Ahmed, N. (2005). Advanced glycation endproducts—Role in pathology of diabetic complications. *Diabetes Research and Clinical Practice*, *67*(1), 3–21. http://dx.doi.org/10.1016/j.diabres.2004.09.004.

Akihiro, A., Masuda, T., Misao, O., Ryosuke, S., Michitaka, K., Daisuke, K., … Junya, A. (2014). Abstract 12859: Increased physical activity prevents the progress of left ventricular hypertrophy via reducing advanced glycation end-products in patients with hypertension circulation. *Physical Activity Prevents the Progress of Left Ventricular*, *130*(2).

Allmen, E. U., Koch, M., Fritz, G., & Legler, D. F. (2008). V domain of RAGE interacts with AGEs on prostate carcinoma cells. *Prostate*, *68*(7), 748–758. http://dx.doi.org/10.1002/pros.20736.

Ames, J. M. (2008). Determination of N epsilon-(carboxymethyl)lysine in foods and related systems. *Annals of the New York Academy of Sciences*, *1126*, 20–24. http://dx.doi.org/10.1196/annals.1433.030.

Ansari, N. A., & Raseed, Z. (2008). Non-enzymatic glycation of proteins: From diabetes to cancer. *Biomedical Chemistry*, *3*(4), 335–342.

Ansari, N. A., & Rasheed, Z. (2010). Non-enzymatic glycation of proteins: From diabetes to cancer. *Biomeditsinskaya Khimiya*, *56*(2), 168–178.

Aseervatham, G. S., Sivasudha, T., Jeyadevi, R., & Arul Ananth, D. (2013). Environmental factors and unhealthy lifestyle influence oxidative stress in humans—An overview. *Environmental Science and Pollution Research International*, *20*(7), 4356–4369. http://dx.doi.org/10.1007/s11356-013-1748-0.

Bansal, S., Siddarth, M., Chawla, D., Banerjee, B. D., Madhu, S. V., & Tripathi, A. K. (2012). Advanced glycation end products enhance reactive oxygen and nitrogen species generation in neutrophils in vitro. *Molecular and Cellular Biochemistry*, *361*(1–2), 289–296. http://dx.doi.org/10.1007/s11010-011-1114-9.

Bao, J. M., He, M. Y., Liu, Y. W., Lu, Y. J., Hong, Y. Q., Luo, H. H., … Jiang, Y. (2015). AGE/RAGE/Akt pathway contributes to prostate cancer cell proliferation by promoting Rb phosphorylation and degradation. *American Journal of Cancer Research*, *5*(5), 1741–1750.

Barea, F., & Bonatto, D. (2008). Relationships among carbohydrate intermediate metabolites and DNA damage and repair in yeast from a systems biology perspective. *Mutation Research*, *642*(1–2), 43–56. http://dx.doi.org/10.1016/j.mrfmmm.2008.04.003.

Baynes, J. W. (2001). The role of AGEs in aging: Causation or correlation. *Experimental Gerontology*, *36*(9), 1527–1537.

Boor, P., Celec, P., Behuliak, M., Grancic, P., Kebis, A., Kukan, M., … Sebekova, K. (2009). Regular moderate exercise reduces advanced glycation and ameliorates early diabetic nephropathy in obese Zucker rats. *Metabolism, 58*(11), 1669–1677. http://dx.doi.org/10.1016/j.metabol.2009.05.025S0026-0495(09)00224-8.

Cerami, C., Founds, H., Nicholl, I., Mitsuhashi, T., Giordano, D., Vanpatten, S., … Cerami, A. (1997). Tobacco smoke is a source of toxic reactive glycation products. *Proceedings of the National Academy of Sciences of the United States of America, 94*(25), 13915–13920.

Chang, T., & Wu, L. (2006). Methylglyoxal, oxidative stress, and hypertension. *Canadian Journal of Physiology and Pharmacology, 84*(12), 1229–1238. http://dx.doi.org/10.1139/y06-077.

Cho, S. J., Roman, G., Yeboah, F., & Konishi, Y. (2007). The road to advanced glycation end products: A mechanistic perspective. *Current Medicinal Chemistry, 14*(15), 1653–1671.

Dato, S., Crocco, P., D'Aquila, P., de Rango, F., Bellizzi, D., Rose, G., & Passarino, G. (2013). Exploring the role of genetic variability and lifestyle in oxidative stress response for healthy aging and longevity. *International Journal of Molecular Sciences, 14*(8), 16443–16472. http://dx.doi.org/10.3390/ijms140816443.

de Arriba, S. G., Loske, C., Meiners, I., Fleischer, G., Lobisch, M., Wessel, K., … Munch, G. (2003). Advanced glycation endproducts induce changes in glucose consumption, lactate production, and ATP levels in SH-SY5Y neuroblastoma cells by a redox-sensitive mechanism. *Journal of Cerebral Blood Flow and Metabolism, 23*(11), 1307–1313. http://dx.doi.org/10.1097/01.WCB.0000090622.86921.0E.

Desai, K. M., Chang, T., Wang, H., Banigesh, A., Dhar, A., Liu, J., … Wu, L. (2010). Oxidative stress and aging: Is methylglyoxal the hidden enemy? *Canadian Journal of Physiology and Pharmacology, 88*(3), 273–284. http://dx.doi.org/10.1139/Y10-001.

Duran-Jimenez, B., Dobler, D., Moffatt, S., Rabbani, N., Streuli, C. H., Thornalley, P. J., … Gardiner, N. J. (2009). Advanced glycation end products in extracellular matrix proteins contribute to the failure of sensory nerve regeneration in diabetes. *Diabetes, 58*(12), 2893–2903. http://dx.doi.org/10.2337/db09-0320.

Ekelund, U., Ward, H. A., Norat, T., Luan, J., May, A. M., Weiderpass, E., … Riboli, E. (2015). Physical activity and all-cause mortality across levels of overall and abdominal adiposity in European men and women: The European prospective investigation into cancer and nutrition study (EPIC). *The American Journal of Cancer Research, 101*, 613–621.

Elangovan, I., Thirugnanam, S., Chen, A., Zheng, G., Bosland, M. C., Kajdacsy-Balla, A., & Gnanasekar, M. (2012). Targeting receptor for advanced glycation end products (RAGE) expression induces apoptosis and inhibits prostate tumor growth. *Biochemical and Biophysical Research Communications, 417*(4), 1133–1138. http://dx.doi.org/10.1016/j.bbrc.2011.12.060. S0006-291X(11)02269-8 [pii].

Feairheller, D. L., Park, J. Y., Sturgeon, K. M., Williamson, S. T., Diaz, K. M., Veerabhadrappa, P., & Brown, M. D. (2011). Racial differences in oxidative stress and inflammation: In vitro and in vivo. *Clinical and Translational Science, 4*(1), 32–37. http://dx.doi.org/10.1111/j.1752-8062.2011.00264.x.

Fisher, G., Alvarez, J. A., Ellis, A. C., Granger, W. M., Ovalle, F., Man, C. D., … Gower, B. A. (2012). Race differences in the association of oxidative stress with insulin sensitivity in African- and European-American women. *Obesity (Silver Spring), 20*(5), 972–977. http://dx.doi.org/10.1038/oby.2011.355.

Foster, D., Spruill, L., Walter, K. R., Nogueira, L. M., Fedarovich, H., Turner, R. Y., … Turner, D. P. (2014). AGE metabolites: A biomarker linked to cancer disparity? *Cancer Epidemiology, Biomarkers & Prevention, 23*(10), 2186–2191. http://dx.doi.org/10.1158/1055-9965.epi-14-0564.

Grote, V. A., Nieters, A., Kaaks, R., Tjonneland, A., Roswall, N., Overvad, K., … Rohrmann, S. (2012). The associations of advanced glycation end products and its soluble receptor with pancreatic cancer risk: A case-control study within the prospective EPIC cohort. *Cancer Epidemiology, Biomarkers & Prevention, 21*(4), 619–628. http://dx.doi.org/10.1158/1055-9965.EPI-11-1139.

Guimaraes, E. L., Empsen, C., Geerts, A., & van Grunsven, L. A. (2010). Advanced glycation end products induce production of reactive oxygen species via the activation of NADPH oxidase in murine hepatic stellate cells. *Journal of Hepatology, 52*(3), 389–397. http://dx.doi.org/10.1016/j.jhep.2009.12.007. S0168-8278(09)00808-3 [pii].

Han, L., Li, L., Li, B., Zhao, D., Li, Y., Xu, Z., & Liu, G. (2013). Review of the characteristics of food-derived and endogenous ne-carboxymethyllysine. *Journal of Food Protection, 76*(5), 912–918. http://dx.doi.org/10.4315/0362-028X.JFP-12-472.

Hayashi, N., George, J., Takeuchi, M., Fukumura, A., Toshikuni, N., Arisawa, T., & Tsutsumi, M. (2013). Acetaldehyde-derived advanced glycation end-products promote alcoholic liver disease. *PLoS One, 8(7)*, e70034. PMID23922897.

Ishibashi, Y., Matsui, T., Takeuchi, M., & Yamagishi, S. (2013). Metformin inhibits advanced glycation end products (AGEs)-induced growth and VEGF expression in MCF-7 breast cancer cells by suppressing AGEs receptor expression via AMP-activated protein kinase. *Hormone and Metabolic Research, 45*(5), 387–390. http://dx.doi.org/10.1055/s-0032-1331204.

Jiao, L., Stolzenberg-Solomon, R., Zimmerman, T. P., Duan, Z., Chen, L., Kahle, L., … Sinha, R. (2015). Dietary consumption of advanced glycation end products and pancreatic cancer in the prospective NIH-AARP diet and health study. *American Journal of Clinical Nutrition, 101*(1), 126–134. http://dx.doi.org/10.3945/ajcn.114.098061.

Kalousová, M., Zima, T., Popov, P., Spacek, P., Braun, M., Soukupová, J., … Kientsch-Engel, R. (2004). Advanced glycation end-products in patients with chronic alcohol misuse. *Alcohol Alcohol, 39(4)*, 316–320. PMID 15208163.

Kasznicki, J., Sliwinska, A., & Drzewoski, J. (2014). Metformin in cancer prevention and therapy. *Annals of Translational Medicine, 2*(6), 57. http://dx.doi.org/10.3978/j.issn.2305-5839.2014.06.01.

Kim, J. Y., Park, H. K., Yoon, J. S., Kim, S. J., Kim, E. S., Ahn, K. S., … Lee, Y. Y. (2008). Advanced glycation end product (AGE)-induced proliferation of HEL cells via receptor for AGE-related signal pathways. *International Journal of Oncology, 33*(3), 493–501.

Kinseth, M. A., Jia, Z., Rahmatpanah, F., Sawyers, A., Sutton, M., Wang-Rodriguez, J., … McGuire, K. L. (2014). Expression differences between African American and Caucasian prostate cancer tissue reveals that stroma is the site of aggressive changes. *International Journal of Cancer, 134*(1), 81–91. http://dx.doi.org/10.1002/ijc.28326.

Korwar, A. M., Bhonsle, H. S., Chougale, A. D., Kote, S. S., Gawai, K. R., Ghole, V. S., … Kulkarni, M. J. (2012). Analysis of AGE modified proteins and RAGE expression in HER2/neu negative invasive ductal carcinoma. *Biochemical and Biophysical Research Communications, 419*(3), 490–494. http://dx.doi.org/10.1016/j.bbrc.2012.02.039.

Li, S. Y., Sigmon, V. K., Babcock, S. A., & Ren, J. (2007). Advanced glycation endproduct induces ROS accumulation, apoptosis, MAP kinase activation and nuclear O-GlcNAcylation in human cardiac myocytes. *Life Sciences, 80*(11), 1051–1056. http://dx.doi.org/10.1016/j.lfs.2006.11.035.

Martin, D. N., Starks, A. M., & Ambs, S. (2013). Biological determinants of health disparities in prostate cancer. *Current Opinion in Oncology, 25*(3), 235–241. http://dx.doi.org/10.1097/CCO.0b013e32835eb5d1.

Morita, M., Yano, S., Yamaguchi, T., & Sugimoto, T. (2013). Advanced glycation end products-induced reactive oxygen species generation is partly through NF-kappa B activation in human aortic endothelial cells. *Journal of Diabetes and Its Complications, 27*(1), 11–15. http://dx.doi.org/10.1016/j.jdiacomp.2012.07.006. S1056-8727(12) 00227-9 [pii].

Morris, A. A., Zhao, L., Patel, R. S., Jones, D. P., Ahmed, Y., Stoyanova, N., … Quyyumi, A. A. (2012). Differences in systemic oxidative stress based on race and the metabolic syndrome: The Morehouse and Emory Team up to Eliminate Health Disparities (META-Health) study. *Metabolic Syndrome and Related Disorders, 10*(4), 252–259. http://dx.doi.org/10.1089/met.2011.0117.

Nicholl, I. D., & Bucala, R. (1998). Advanced glycation endproducts and cigarette smoking. *Cellular and Molecular Biology (Noisy-le-Grand, France), 44*(7), 1025–1033.

Nomoto, K., Yagi, M., Arita, S., Ogura, M., & Yonei, Y. (2012). Skin accumulation of advanced glycation end products and lifestyle behaviors in Japanese. *Anti-Aging Medicine, 6*, 165–173.

Park, N. J., & Kang, D. H. (2013). Inflammatory cytokine levels and breast cancer risk factors: Racial differences of healthy Caucasian and African American women. *Oncology Nursing Forum, 40*(5), 490–500. http://dx.doi.org/10.1188/13.ONF.40-05AP.

Peppa, M., Uribarri, J., & Vlassara, H. (2008). Aging and glycoxidant stress. *Hormones (Athens, Greece), 7*(2), 123–132.

Powell, I. J., & Bollig-Fischer, A. (2013). Minireview: The molecular and genomic basis for prostate cancer health disparities. *Molecular Endocrinology, 27*(6), 879–891. http://dx.doi.org/10.1210/me.2013-1039.

Pulito, C., Sanli, T., Rana, P., Muti, P., Blandino, G., & Strano, S. (2013). Metformin: On ongoing journey across diabetes, cancer therapy and prevention. *Metabolites, 3*(4), 1051–1075. http://dx.doi.org/10.3390/metabo3041051.

Rahbar, S. (2007). Novel inhibitors of glycation and AGE formation. *Cell Biochemistry and Biophysics, 48*(2–3), 147–157. doi: CBB:48:2-3:147 [pii].

Reams, R. R., Agrawal, D., Davis, M. B., Yoder, S., Odedina, F. T., Kumar, N., … Soliman, K. F. (2009). Microarray comparison of prostate tumor gene expression in African-American and Caucasian American males: A pilot project study. *Infectious Agents and Cancer, 4*(Suppl. 1), S3. http://dx.doi.org/10.1186/1750-9378-4-S1-S3.

Riehl, A., Nemeth, J., Angel, P., & Hess, J. (2009). The receptor RAGE: Bridging inflammation and cancer. *Cell Communication and Signaling, 7*, 12. http://dx.doi.org/10.1186/1478-811X-7-12. 1478-811X-7-12 [pii].

Rodriguez-Teja, M., Gronau, J. H., Breit, C., Zhang, Y. Z., Minamidate, A., Caley, M. P., … Sturge, J. (2014). AGE-modified basement membrane cooperates with Endo180 to promote epithelial cell invasiveness and decrease prostate cancer survival. *Journal of Pathology, 235*, 581–592. http://dx.doi.org/10.1002/path.4485.

Rojas, A., Gonzalez, I., Morales, E., Perez-Castro, R., Romero, J., & Figueroa, H. (2011). Diabetes and cancer: Looking at the multiligand/RAGE axis. *World Journal of Diabetes, 2*(7), 108–113. http://dx.doi.org/10.4239/wjd.v2.i7.108.

Rojas, A., Mercadal, E., Figueroa, H., & Morales, M. A. (2008). Advanced glycation and ROS: A link between diabetes and heart failure. *Current Vascular Pharmacology, 6*(1), 44–51.

Rose, A. E., Satagopan, J. M., Oddoux, C., Zhou, Q., Xu, R., Olshen, A. B., … Osman, I. (2010). Copy number and gene expression differences between African American and Caucasian American prostate cancer. *Journal of Translational Medicine, 8*, 70. http://dx.doi.org/10.1186/1479-5876-8-70.

Salama, M. E., El-Damarawi, M. A., & Salama, A. F. (2013). A comparison between the impact of two different exercise protocols on advanced glycation end products in type 2 diabetic rats. *Life Science Journal, 10*(3), 860–869.

Sharaf, H., Matou-Nasri, S., Wang, Q., Rabhan, Z., Al-Eidi, H., Al Abdulrahman, A., & Ahmed, N. (2015). Advanced glycation endproducts increase proliferation, migration and invasion of the breast cancer cell line MDA-MB-231. *Biochimica et Biophysica Acta*, *1852*(3), 429–441. http://dx.doi.org/10.1016/j.bbadis.2014.12.009.

Shimomoto, T., Luo, Y., Ohmori, H., Chihara, Y., Fujii, K., Sasahira, T., … Kuniyasu, H. (2012). Advanced glycation end products (AGE) induce the receptor for AGE in the colonic mucosa of azoxymethane-injected Fischer 344 rats fed with a high-linoleic acid and high-glucose diet. *Journal of Gastroenterology*, *47*(10), 1073–1083. http://dx.doi.org/10.1007/s00535-012-0572-5.

Singh, R., Barden, A., Mori, T., & Beilin, L. (2001). Advanced glycation end-products: A review. *Diabetologia*, *44*(2), 129–146. http://dx.doi.org/10.1007/s001250051591.

Sparvero, L. J., Asafu-Adjei, D., Kang, R., Tang, D., Amin, N., Im, J., … Lotze, M. T. (2009). RAGE (receptor for advanced glycation endproducts), RAGE ligands, and their role in cancer and inflammation. *Journal of Translational Medicine*, 7, 17. http://dx.doi.org/10.1186/1479-5876-7-17.

Stirban, A., Negrean, M., Gotting, C., Uribarri, J., Gawlowski, T., Stratmann, B., … Tschoepe, D. (2008). Dietary advanced glycation endproducts and oxidative stress: In vivo effects on endothelial function and adipokines. *Annals of the New York Academy of Sciences*, *1126*, 276–279. http://dx.doi.org/10.1196/annals.1433.042. 1126/1/276 [pii].

Stirban, A., Negrean, M., Stratmann, B., Gawlowski, T., Horstmann, T., Gotting, C., … Tschoepe, D. (2006). Benfotiamine prevents macro- and microvascular endothelial dysfunction and oxidative stress following a meal rich in advanced glycation end products in individuals with type 2 diabetes. *Diabetes Care*, *29*(9), 2064–2071. http://dx.doi.org/10.2337/dc06-0531. 29/9/2064 [pii].

Suissa, S., & Azoulay, L. (2014). Metformin and cancer: Mounting evidence against an association. *Diabetes Care*, *37*(7), 1786–1788. http://dx.doi.org/10.2337/dc14-0500.

Thornalley, P. J. (2003a). The enzymatic defence against glycation in health, disease and therapeutics: A symposium to examine the concept. *Biochemical Society Transactions*, *31*(Pt 6), 1341–1342. http://dx.doi.org/10.1042/bst0311341.

Thornalley, P. J. (2003b). Protecting the genome: Defence against nucleotide glycation and emerging role of glyoxalase I overexpression in multidrug resistance in cancer chemotherapy. *Biochemical Society Transactions*, *31*(Pt 6), 1372–1377. http://dx.doi.org/10.1042/bst0311372.

Thornalley, P. J. (2008). Protein and nucleotide damage by glyoxal and methylglyoxal in physiological systems—Role in ageing and disease. *Drug Metabolism and Drug Interactions*, *23*(1–2), 125–150.

Turner, D. P. (2015). Advanced glycation end-products: A biological consequence of lifestyle contributing to cancer disparity. *Cancer Research*, *75*(10), 1925–1929. http://dx.doi.org/10.1158/0008-5472.can-15-0169.

Uribarri, J., Cai, W., Peppa, M., Goodman, S., Ferrucci, L., Striker, G., & Vlassara, H. (2007). Circulating glycotoxins and dietary advanced glycation endproducts: Two links to inflammatory response, oxidative stress, and aging. *Journals of Gerontology. Series A, Biological Sciences and Medical Sciences*, *62*(4), 427–433.

Uribarri, J., Cai, W., Sandu, O., Peppa, M., Goldberg, T., & Vlassara, H. (2005). Diet-derived advanced glycation end products are major contributors to the body's AGE pool and induce inflammation in healthy subjects. *Annals of the New York Academy of Sciences*, *1043*, 461–466. http://dx.doi.org/10.1196/annals.1333.052. 1043/1/461 [pii].

Uribarri, J., Woodruff, S., Goodman, S., Cai, W., Chen, X., Pyzik, R., … Vlassara, H. (2010). Advanced glycation end products in foods and a practical guide to their reduction in the diet. *Journal of the American Dietetic Association*, *110*(6), 911–916 e912. http://dx.doi.org/10.1016/j.jada.2010.03.018. S0002-8223(10)00238-5 [pii].

van Heijst, J. W., Niessen, H. W., Hoekman, K., & Schalkwijk, C. G. (2005). Advanced glycation end products in human cancer tissues: Detection of Nepsilon-(carboxymethyl)lysine and argpyrimidine. *Annals of the New York Academy of Sciences, 1043*, 725–733. http://dx.doi.org/10.1196/annals.1333.084. 1043/1/725 [pii].

Vlassara, H. (2005). Advanced glycation in health and disease: Role of the modern environment. *Annals of the New York Academy of Sciences, 1043*, 452–460. http://dx.doi.org/10.1196/annals.1333.051. 1043/1/452 [pii].

Wautier, M. P., Chappey, O., Corda, S., Stern, D. M., Schmidt, A. M., & Wautier, J. L. (2001). Activation of NADPH oxidase by AGE links oxidant stress to altered gene expression via RAGE. *American Journal of Physiology. Endocrinology and Metabolism, 280*(5), E685–E694.

Wautier, J. L., & Schmidt, A. M. (2004). Protein glycation: A firm link to endothelial cell dysfunction. *Circulation Research, 95*(3), 233–238. http://dx.doi.org/10.1161/01.RES.0000137876.28454.64.

Weyemi, U., Redon, C. E., Parekh, P. R., Dupuy, C., & Bonner, W. M. (2013). NADPH oxidases NOXs and DUOXs as putative targets for cancer therapy. *Anti-Cancer Agents in Medicinal Chemistry, 13*(3), 502–514.

Wright, K. J., Thomas, M. M., Betik, A. C., Belke, D., & Hepple, R. T. (2014). Exercise training initiated in late middle age attenuates cardiac fibrosis and advanced glycation end-product accumulation in senescent rats. *Experimental Gerontology, 50*, 9–18. http://dx.doi.org/10.1016/j.exger.2013.11.006.

Wuenschell, G. E., Tamae, D., Cercillieux, A., Yamanaka, R., Yu, C., & Termini, J. (2010). Mutagenic potential of DNA glycation: Miscoding by (R)- and (S)-N(2)-(1-carboxyethyl)-2′-deoxyguanosine. *Biochemistry, 49*(9), 1814–1821. http://dx.doi.org/10.1021/bi901924b.

Yamagishi, S., Nakamura, K., Matsui, T., Ueda, S., Fukami, K., & Okuda, S. (2008). Agents that block advanced glycation end product (AGE)-RAGE (receptor for AGEs)-oxidative stress system: A novel therapeutic strategy for diabetic vascular complications. *Expert Opinion on Investigational Drugs, 17*(7), 983–996. http://dx.doi.org/10.1517/13543784.17.7.983.

Yang, S., Pinney, S. M., Mallick, P., Ho, S. M., Bracken, B., & Wu, T. (2015). Impact of oxidative stress biomarkers and carboxymethyllysine (an advanced glycation end product) on prostate cancer: A prospective study. *Clinical Genitourinary Cancer, 13*(5), e347–e351. http://dx.doi.org/10.1016/j.clgc.2015.04.004.

Yao, D., & Brownlee, M. (2010). Hyperglycemia-induced reactive oxygen species increase expression of the receptor for advanced glycation end products (RAGE) and RAGE ligands. *Diabetes, 59*(1), 249–255. http://dx.doi.org/10.2337/db09-0801.

Yoshikawa, T., Miyazaki, A., & Fujimoto, S. (2009). Decrease in serum levels of advanced glycation end-products by short-term lifestyle modification in non-diabetic middle-aged females. *Medical Science Monitor, 15*(6), PH65–PH73.

CHAPTER TWO

# Disparities in Obesity, Physical Activity Rates, and Breast Cancer Survival

M.E. Ford*,†,[1], G. Magwood*, E.T. Brown‡, K. Cannady*,†, M. Gregoski§, K.D. Knight*,†, L.L. Peterson¶, R. Kramer*, A. Evans-Knowell||, D.P. Turner*,†

*Medical University of South Carolina, Charleston, SC, United States
†Hollings Cancer Center, Medical University of South Carolina, Charleston, SC, United States
‡Morehouse School of Medicine, Atlanta, GA, United States
§Campbell University, Buies Creek, NC, United States
¶Washington University School of Medicine, St. Louis, MO, United States
||South Carolina State University, Orangeburg, SC, United States
[1]Corresponding author: e-mail address: fordmar@musc.edu

## Contents



*Advances in Cancer Research*, Volume 133
ISSN 0065-230X
http://dx.doi.org/10.1016/bs.acr.2016.08.002

## Abstract

The significantly higher breast cancer (BCa) mortality rates of African-American (AA) women compared to non-Hispanic (NHW) white women constitute a major US health disparity. Investigations have primarily focused on biological differences in tumors to explain more aggressive forms of BCa in AA women. The biology of tumors cannot be modified, yet lifestyle changes can mitigate their progression and recurrence. AA communities have higher percentages of obesity than NHWs and exhibit inefficient access to care, low socioeconomic status, and reduced education levels. Such factors are associated with limited healthy food options and sedentary activity. AA women have the highest prevalence of obesity than any other racial/ethnic/gender group in the United States. The social ecological model (SEM) is a conceptual framework on which interventions could be developed to reduce obesity. The SEM includes intrapersonal factors, interpersonal factors, organizational relationships, and community/institutional policies that are more effective in behavior modification than isolation from the participants' environmental context. Implementation of SEM-based interventions in AA communities could positively modify lifestyle behaviors, which could also serve as a powerful tool in reducing risk of BCa, BCa progression, and BCa recurrence in populations of AA women.

## 1. INTRODUCTION

Breast cancer (BCa) is the second leading cause of new cancer cases in the United States. Early detection and more effective treatments have resulted in approximately 3.5 million BCa survivors now living in the United States, thus constituting a major public health concern. The long-term health and well-being of BCa survivors is of interest to the scientific community as lifestyle behaviors such as obesity, poor diet, and physical inactivity may have distinct molecular consequences for BCa recurrence. The purpose of this chapter is to carefully explicate these relationships.

## 2. LITERATURE REVIEW AND SYNTHESIS

### 2.1 Disparities in Breast Cancer Mortality Rates in the United States

Breast cancer accounts for 19% of cancer deaths in African Americans (AA; DeSantis et al., 2016). As DeSantis et al. (2016) note, the causes of the disproportionate breast cancer burden experienced by AA women are complex and primarily reflect social and economic disparities as well as biological differences. These authors point out that in 2014, 26% of AAs compared to 10% of non-Hispanic whites (NHWs) had incomes below the federal poverty level. Similarly, in 2014, only 22% of AAs had 4-year college degrees, compared to 36% of NHWs, indicating a higher earning potential and greater likelihood of having adequate health insurance coverage among whites.

These socioeconomic factors are reflected in the presence of disparities in the lifetime probability (%) of developing or dying from invasive breast cancer in 2010–2012 (DeSantis et al., 2016). These data show that AA women had an 11.1% probability of developing breast cancer, as compared to a 13.1% probability among NHW women during the same time period. However, AA women had a 3.3% probability of dying from breast cancer, as compared to a 2.7% probability among NHW women. The increased mortality in AA women is present despite a lower incidence of BCa. The 5-year relative survival rate is lower in AA women with BCa than for white women, for every stage of diagnosis, as shown below (American Cancer Society, 2016a; DeSantis et al., 2016; Fig. 1).

As McCarthy, Yang, and Armstrong (2015) note, the racial disparity in BCa mortality has widened over the past 30 years. Racial/ethnic disparities in 5-year relative survival rates are believed to be due primarily to differences

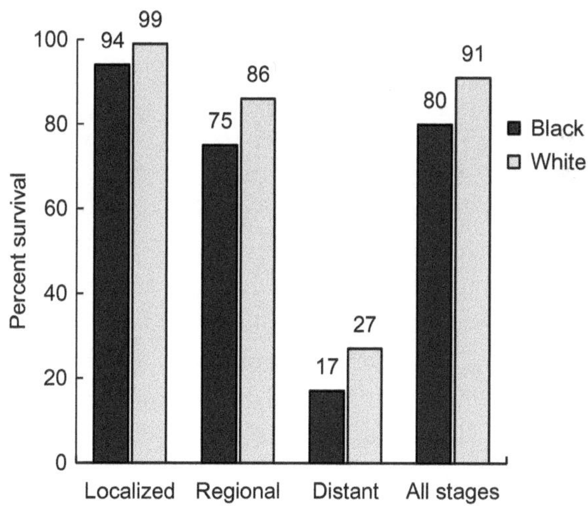


**Fig. 1** Female breast cancer survival rates in the United States, based on patients diagnosed between 2005 and 2011 and followed through 2012. *Adapted from American Cancer Society (2016a). Cancer facts & figures for African Americans 2016–2018. Atlanta: American Cancer Society.*

in timely access to appropriate BCa screening, diagnosis, and treatment. Factors affecting access to care include insurance coverage, transportation, and ability to afford recommended medications. AA women tend to be diagnosed with BCa at later stages than NHW women, indicative of the receipt of fewer mammograms, longer intervals between mammographic screening and untimely follow-up of abnormal BCa screening results (DeSantis et al., 2016; Hoffman et al., 2011; Press, Carrasquillo, Sciacca, & Giardina, 2008; Smith-Bindman et al., 2006) As Reeder-Hayes, Wheeler, and Mayer (2015) note, disparities in cancer care extend to survivorship care, where minority women receive endocrine therapy at lower rates than white women (Reeder-Hayes et al., 2015). Previous studies have demonstrated that when AAs receive cancer treatments similar to those received by NHWs, their cancer mortality outcomes are comparable (Bach et al., 2002; Komenaka et al., 2010). Along similar lines, Daly and Olopade (2015) point to reduced access to care for BCa screening and treatment, coupled with a more aggressive form of BCa, as major contributors to the racial disparity in BCa survival between AA and white women.

The increasing disparity in BCa mortality between AA and NHW women is not due to socioeconomic factors alone. AA women are also more likely to be diagnosed with aggressive BCa tumor subtypes. According to DeSantis et al. (2016), the prevalence of estrogen receptor-negative, progesterone receptor-negative, and human epidermal growth factor receptor 2-negative ("triple-negative") BCa is 22% in AA women and only 10–12% among women from other racial/ethnic backgrounds. Among premenopausal AA women, the prevalence of triple-negative BCa is even higher (Danforth, 2013). AA women are also more likely than other women to be diagnosed with basal-like breast tumors, which are associated with poorer survival rates than other breast tumor subtypes (Warner et al., 2015).

Similarly, Warner et al. (2015) note that BCa subtypes may help to account for racial/ethnic differences in survival. These investigators analyzed prospective cohort data from women diagnosed with Stages I–III BCa at National Comprehensive Cancer Network centers between January 2000 and December 2007 with survival follow-up through December 2009. The cases (533 Asian Americans; 1122 Hispanics; 1345 African Americans; and 14,268 non-Hispanic whites) were stratified by subtype (luminal A-like, luminal B-like, human epidermal growth factor receptor 2 (HER2) subtype, and triple-negative). According to the results, AA women were more likely to die from luminal A-like and luminal B-like tumors than NHW women. No disparities were observed for HER2 or triple-negative subtypes, although

Asian American and Hispanic women were less likely to die as a result of BCa compared to NHW women.

D'Arcy et al. (2015) examined gene expression breast tumor data from 108 European American (EA) women and 57 AA women and found that AA women have higher mortality rates with luminal A breast cancers, which generally have a more favorable prognosis. These results were corroborated by Ma et al. (2013) who investigated the disparity in BCa mortality, stratified by BCa subtype (ER, PR, and HER2 status). In a sample of 1204 women (523 African Americans and 681 European Americans), older AA women (ages 50–64 years) diagnosed with luminal A invasive BCa were found to have a higher mortality risk than EA women in the same age group who were diagnosed with the same BCa subtype. These investigators argue that disparities in mortality related to luminal A BCas, rather than disparities in mortality related to triple-negative BCa, drive the observed black–white difference in BCa mortality. Conversely, Tao, Gomez, Keegan, Kurian, and Clarke (2015) evaluated data from 93,760 EA women and 9738 AA women and discovered that, among those with luminal A or triple-negative BCa, AA women had higher mortality rates.

To assess the degree to which biological differences (in addition to treatment or health care access issues) may contribute to these mortality differences, D'Arcy et al. (2015) evaluated the expression of race- and survival-associated genes in normal tissue and BCa tumor tissue of AA and EA women. These investigators found that six genes (ACOX2, MUC1, CRYBB2, PSPH, SQLE, and TYMS) were expressed differentially in the luminal A breast cancers of these two groups of women and were linked with survival (HR $<0.08$; HR $>1.25$). For all six genes, the tumors in the AA women showed higher rates of expression of poor prognosis genes (CRYBB2, PSPH, SQLE, and TYMS) and lower rates of expression of good prognosis genes (ACOX2 and MUC1). In addition, two of the poor prognosis genes (CRYBB2 and PSPH) had higher expression in the normal tissue of AA women than EA women. These findings demonstrate the importance of assessing potential biological contributors to BCa mortality disparities.

In the Warner et al. (2015) study, a racial disparity was seen in death due to BCa. Specifically, (a) disparities in mortality outcomes persisted for AAs even after controlling for stage at diagnosis, tumor characteristics, and body mass index (BMI); (b) AA women were most likely to be diagnosed with triple-negative tumors. However, the greatest survival disparities were evident among AA women with luminal tumors, as compared to NHW women with luminal tumors. The highest mortality rates among AAs were seen in the first 2 years postdiagnosis with ER-positive tumors (Warner et al., 2015). This differential mortality rate may be at least partially explained by AAs' delays in initiation, or incomplete receipt of BCa surgery, chemotherapy, or hormonal therapy (Warner et al., 2015).

As there are currently no FDA approved targeted therapies for triple-negative breast tumors, women diagnosed with this form of BCa tend to have a poorer prognosis than other women. While some recent studies have identified genes that may be related to the prevalence of triple-negative BCa in AA women, other studies show that lifestyle factors more common among AA women, such as obesity, having a high number of children, age at first pregnancy, as well as low rates of breastfeeding, may contribute to an increased risk for triple-negative BCa (Dietze, Sistrunk, Miranda-Carboni, O'Regan, & Seewaldt, 2015; Palmer et al., 2014; Phipps et al., 2011; Yang et al., 2007).

Importantly, the racial disparity in BCa mortality rates continues to widen in the United States. In fact, in a comparison of BCa death rates between AAs and NHWs from 2008 to 2012, DeSantis et al. showed the following data: American Cancer Society (2016a) and DeSantis et al. (2016) (Table 1).

As shown in Fig. 2, the disparity gap in BCa mortality between AAs and NHWs remains fairly wide.

The continued gap in BCa mortality rates between AAs and NHWs is attributed to a smaller rate of decrease in BCa mortality rates over time for AA women (American Cancer Society, 2016a). Interestingly, the previously referenced cohort data from Warner et al. (2015) showed that BMI, in addition to breast tumor subtype, contributed to racial differences in BCa survival. While the biological bases of BCa disparities may not be easily modified, the contributions of BMI to racial and ethnic disparities in BCa mortality represent a modifiable behavioral target that could be positively changed through effective behavioral lifestyle interventions.

**Table 1** Comparison of Female Breast Cancer Mortality Rates for African Americans (AAs) and Non-Hispanic Whites (NHWs), United States, 2008–2012

| Breast Cancer Mortality Rates | | | |
|---|---|---|---|
| **AA Mortality Rate** | **NHW Mortality Rate** | **Absolute Difference** | **Rate Ratio** |
| 31.0 | 21.9 | 9.1 | 1.42 |

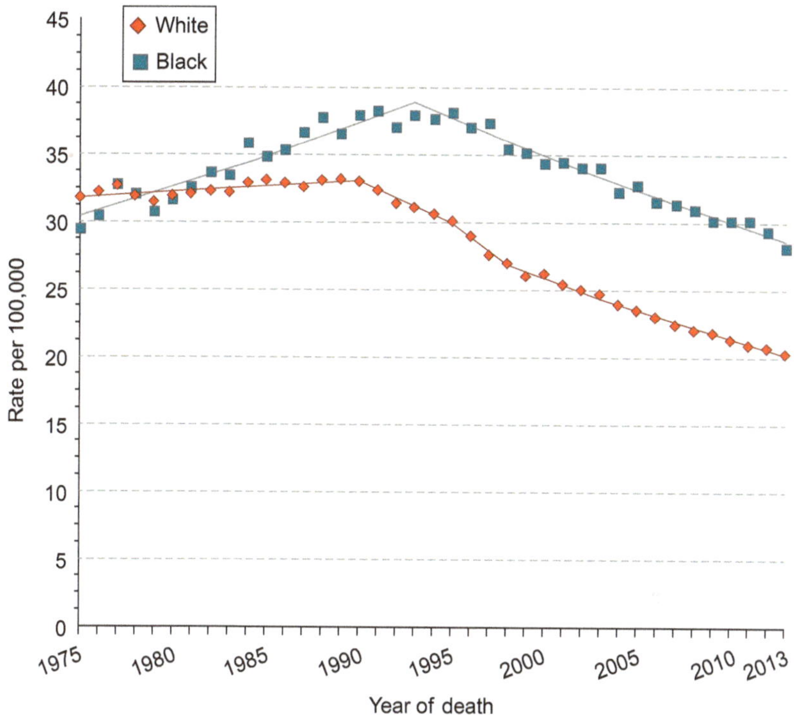


**Fig. 2** Age-adjusted US mortality rates by race/ethnicity, female breast, all ages, 1975–2013. Cancer sites include invasive cases only unless otherwise noted. Rates are per 100,000 and are age-adjusted to the 2000 US Std. Population (19 age groups—Census P25-1130). *Regression lines* are calculated using the Joinpoint Regression Program Version 4.2.0, April 2015 National Cancer Institute. (Fast Stats: An interactive tool for access to SEER cancer statistics. Surveillance Research Program, National Cancer Institute http://seer.cancer.gov/faststats.)

## 2.2 Relationship Between Weight, Physical Activity, and Breast Cancer Recurrence and Mortality

The American Cancer Society (2008) reports that obesity and overweight are associated with 14–20% of all cancer-related deaths. Obesity and overweight increase the risk for BCa in postmenopausal women and may increase the risk in some premenopausal women, particularly ages 35 and over with additional risk factors (American Cancer Society, 2008; Cecchini et al., 2012; Demark-Wahnefried, Campbell, & Hayes, 2012; Fabian, 2012; Pischon, Nothlings, & Boeing, 2008; Renehan, Roberts, & Dive, 2008). Indeed, on page 12 of the seminal report titled "Cancer facts & figures for African Americans 2016–2018", the American Cancer Society states:

*All women can help reduce their risk of breast cancer by avoiding weight gain and obesity (for postmenopausal breast cancer), engaging in regular physical activity, and minimizing alcohol intake.*

***American Cancer Society (2016a)***

Among premenopausal women in the National Surgical Adjuvant Breast and Bowel Project, higher BMI levels were significantly related to increased BCa risk among premenopausal women older than 35 years of age who had additional BCa risk factors (primarily due to a diagnosis of lobular carcinoma in situ) (Cecchini et al., 2012). In a study of 73,542 premenopausal and 103,344 postmenopausal women from 9 European countries, it was discovered that among postmenopausal women who did not take hormone replacement therapy, obese women had a 31% excess risk of developing BCa compared to nonoverweight women (Lahmann et al., 2004). Similar results were found by Morimoto et al. (2002) in a study of 85,917 women in the Women's Health Initiative Observational Study, with participants from 40 clinics in the United States.

## 2.3 Known Biological Mechanisms Link Obesity and Breast Cancer

Emerging research documents the relationship between obesity and BCa etiology and outcomes. Recent investigations suggest that insulin resistance, insulin-like growth factors (IGF-I), and obesity-related inflammatory markers mediate the association between obesity and cancer incidence and mortality (Brown & Simpson, 2012; Costa, Incio, & Soares, 2007; Renehan et al., 2008). It is becoming clear that obesity leads to an increase in circulating insulin and IGF-I, which promotes tumor cell growth.

As Campbell, Foster-Schubert, et al. (2012) and Campbell, Van Patten, et al. (2012) note, overweight/obesity and a sedentary lifestyle significantly increase the risk of BCa. This increased risk may be due primarily to the higher estrogen levels seen in individuals with excess adipose tissue. Higher levels of circulating estrogen are found in women with higher BMIs. Obesity and IGF-I together increase estrogen production in the breast, which significantly increases the risk of BCa and the growth of BCa cells (Brown & Simpson, 2012).

Fortunately, obesity/overweight is a modifiable BCa risk factor. A recent study by Campbell, Van Patten, et al. (2012) demonstrates that among BCa survivors, a 24-week group-based lifestyle intervention modeled after the Diabetes Prevention Program for early stage, BCa survivors produced an average weight loss of $3.8 \pm 5.0$ kg and a decrease in BMI, percent body fat, and waist and hip circumferences at 24 weeks. These strong results were found in women who had already been diagnosed with BCa. While the focus of their study was on women with BCa, the intervention strategies could easily be modified to focus on AA women at risk of developing BCa due to their high rates of obesity.

Indeed, Campbell, Foster-Schubert, et al. (2012) conducted a single-blind, 12-month, randomized controlled trial from 2005 to 2009 with 439 postmenopausal women in the Nutrition and Exercise for Women Trial. Participants, 8% of whom were AA women, were randomly assigned to one of four groups: (1) reduced-calorie weight loss diet, (2) moderate- to vigorous-intensity aerobic exercise; (3) combined reduced-calorie weight loss diet plus moderate- to vigorous-intensity aerobic exercise; or (4) control. Their data show that compared with controls, estrone levels (a natural estrogen) decreased 9.6% with diet alone ($p < 0.001$), decreased 5.5% with exercise alone ($p = 0.01$), and decreased 11.1% with diet plus exercise ($p < 0.001$). Given that high estrogen levels increase the risk of breast cancer, these results highlight the significant potential impact of dietary and physical activity lifestyle changes on BCa risk. In a recent meta-analysis, physical activity has been shown to be protective, reducing the risk of breast cancer compared to women less active, by 22% (Pizot et al., 2016). Obesity can also be successfully treated with lifestyle modifications to lower the risk of developing BCa. Weight loss of 5–10% of body weight that is sustained over several years is needed to lower BCa risk (Eliassen, Colditz, Rosner, Willett, & Hankinson, 2006).

## 2.4 Prevalence of Overweight/Obesity and Physical Inactivity in the United States

Obesity/overweight is a major public health problem in the United States. As shown in a recent report from the *Journal of the American Medical Association*, more than 30% of adults and 17% of youths in the United States are obese, and these prevalence rates have remained stable over the past several years (Ogden, Carroll, Kit, & Flegal, 2014). When obesity and overweight data are combined, 69% of US adults and 21% of US children are obese or overweight (Cecchini et al., 2012; Centers for Disease Control and Prevention (CDC), 2016; Khan et al., 2009). Overweight is defined as a BMI of 25.0–29.9, while obesity is defined as a BMI $\geq 30.0$.

The following prevalence maps highlight the widespread geographic distribution of overweight/obesity prevalence rates across the United States (CDC, 2016). Since 1988, although overweight and obesity prevalence rates have increased among both AAs and NHWs, these rates are significantly higher for African Americans as shown below (National Center for Health Statistics, 2015; Figs. 3–5).

## 2.5 Disparities in Overweight/Obesity and Physical Activity in the United States

Obesity prevalence among AA women is alarming; they have the highest prevalence of obesity than any other racial/ethnic/gender group in the United States (Gaillard, Schuster, & Osei, 2012; James, Pobee, Oxidine, Brown, & Joshi, 2012; Moore-Greene, Gross, Silver, & Perrino, 2012). Less than 20% of AA women have a healthy body weight (Ogden et al., 2006). Even though 70% of AA women report wanting to lose weight and 50% report actively trying to lose weight (Mack et al., 2004), they tend to lose less weight than other women (Kumanyika et al., 2011) and engage in weight loss activities for shorter periods of time.

Large disparities in the prevalence of obesity/overweight are evident across racial, ethnic and socioeconomic status (SES) groups in the United States (Wang & Chen, 2011, 2012). Obesity/overweight occurs with higher prevalence among women, racial/ethnic minorities, and those from a lower

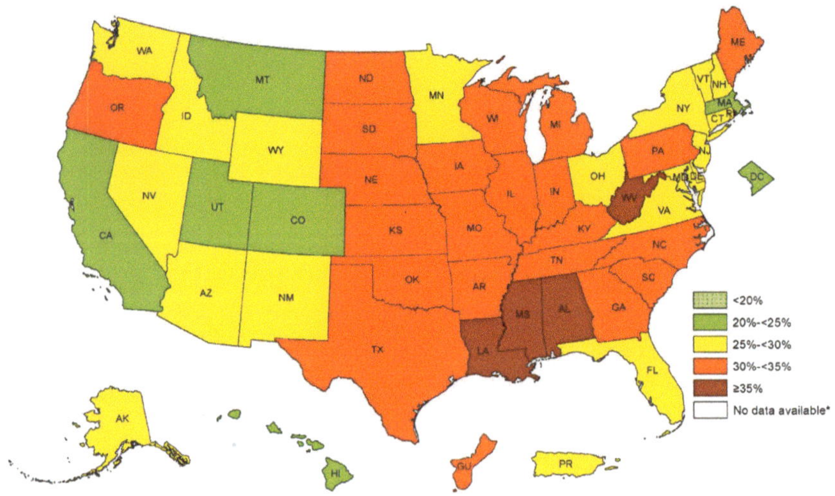


**Fig. 3** Prevalence* of self-reported obesity among US adults by state and territory, BRFSS, 2015. Prevalence estimates reflect BRFSS methodological changes started in 2011. These estimates should not be compared to prevalence estimates before 2011. Sample size <50 or the relative standard error (dividing the standard error by the prevalence) ≥30% (CDC, 2015).

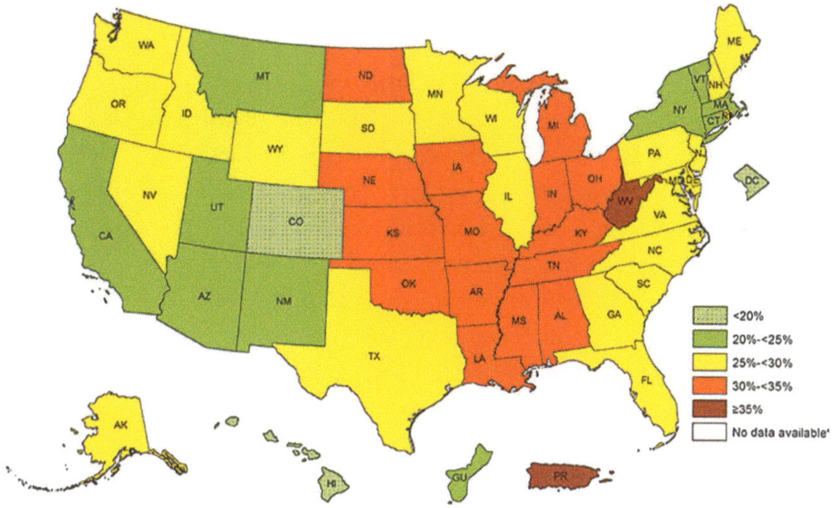


**Fig. 4** Prevalence of self-reported obesity among non-Hispanic White adults by state and territory, BRFSS, 2013–2015. The sample size <50 or the relative standard error (dividing the standard error by the prevalence) ≥30% (CDC, 2015).

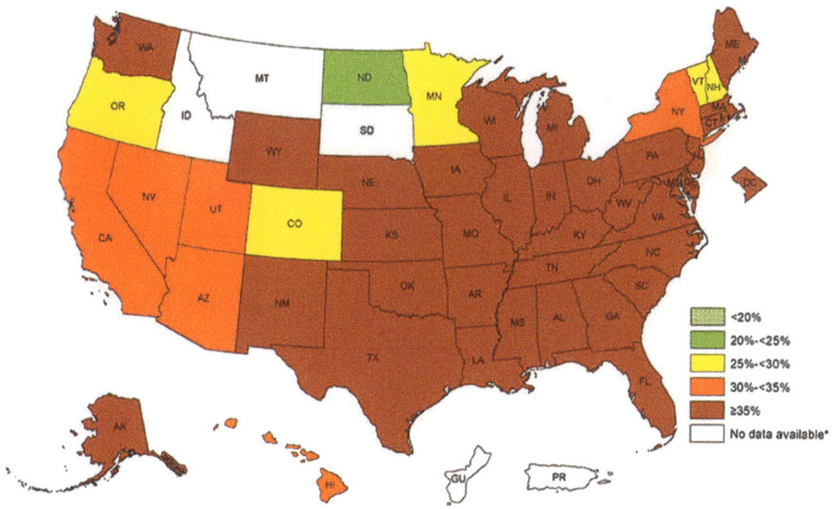


**Fig. 5** Prevalence of self-reported obesity among non-Hispanic black adults by state and territory, BRFSS, 2013–2015. Sample size <50 or the relative standard error (dividing the standard error by the prevalence) ≥30% (CDC, 2015).

SES (Clarke, O'Malley, Johnston, & Schulenberg, 2009; Sauaia & Byers, 2012). For example, Wang and Chen (2012) examined nationally representative data from two sources of survey data, the Continuing Survey of Food Intakes by Individuals and the Diet and Health Knowledge Survey. Data from 4356 adults, ages 20–65 years, were evaluated. Consistent with national data on obesity, these data show that AAs reported the worst average Healthy Eating Index of all racial/ethnic groups ($p<0.05$). However, among participants with a poor diet, those who were female, had greater than a high school education or had comorbidities, were more likely than others to report intention to improve diet ($p<0.05$). Similarly, Coogan, Wise, Cozier, Palmer, and Rosenberg (2012) found that in their sample of 21,457 women ages <55 years in the longitudinal Black Women's Health Study, risk of obesity was lowest among women with college degrees. These findings are significant because they highlight the fact that AA women, who are at risk of developing BCa due to their high BMI, are an ideal focus of weight-reduction interventions.

A recent study of 1280 educated AA women who had at least some college education and who intentionally achieved clinically significant weight loss of at least 10% of body weight showed that 28% of the women maintained ≥10% weight loss for an average of 5.1 years. Women who were successful in maintaining their weight loss were more likely than other women to limit their fat intake, eat breakfast on most days of the week, shun fast food restaurants, take part in moderate to high levels of physical activity, and monitor their weight using a scale (Barnes & Kimbro, 2012).

Thus, national data demonstrate the complex interplay between race/ethnicity and SES in incidence and prevalence of obesity/overweight. These findings show that while race and ethnicity are nonmodifiable factors, obesogenic correlates of low SES, such as education and access to healthy foods and physical activity, are modifiable targets of interventions to reduce obesity/overweight and BCa risk.

Table 2 shows the high rates of obesity and overweight in the United States, with AAs showing significantly higher rates of obesity and overweight compared to the national averages.

Tables 3–8 show that since 1988, AA women have consistently had higher BMI rates than NHW women, even though the obesity rates in both groups decreased from 1988 to 2012 (National Center for Health Statistics, 2015).

**Table 2** Current Obesity and Overweight Rates Among Adults by Race, 2011–2012

| | |
|---|---|
| All adults | 68.5% |
| Race/ethnicity | |
| Black | 76.2% |
| Latino | 77.9% |
| White | 67.2% |

Adapted from Robert Wood Johnson Data: http://stateofobesity.org/disparities/. retrieved September 19, 2016.

**Table 3** Percentage of US Individuals at a Healthy Weight (BMI From 18.5 to 24.9), by Race/Ethnicity, 1988–2012

| | 1988–1994 | 1999–2002 | 2002–2006 | 2009–2012 |
|---|---|---|---|---|
| Non-Hispanic White female | 48.7 | 39.5 | 39.6 | 36.0 |
| Black or African-American female | 29.2 | 21.6 | 19.2 | 16.4 |

Adapted from National Center for Health Statistics (2015). *Health, United States, 2014: With special feature on adults aged 55–64*. http://www.cdc.gov/nchs/data/hus/hus14.pdf#059, Retrieved March 21, 2016.

**Table 4** Percentage of Overweight US Individuals (BMI ≥ 25.0), by Race/Ethnicity, 1988–2012

| | 1988–1994 | 1999–2002 | 2002–2006 | 2009–2012 |
|---|---|---|---|---|
| Non-Hispanic White female | 47.4 | 58.2 | 59.4 | 62.9 |
| Black or African-American female | 66.0 | 76.9 | 79.7 | 82.1 |

Adapted from National Center for Health Statistics (2015). *Health, United States, 2014: With special feature on adults aged 55–64*. http://www.cdc.gov/nchs/data/hus/hus14.pdf#059, Retrieved March 21, 2016.

**Table 5** Percentage of Obese US Individuals (BMI ≥ 30.0), by Race/Ethnicity, 1988–2012

| | 1988–1994 | 1999–2002 | 2002–2006 | 2009–2012 |
|---|---|---|---|---|
| Non-Hispanic White female | 22.7 | 31.3 | 32.2 | 33.5 |
| Black or African-American female | 36.7 | 48.7 | 53.2 | 57.6 |

Adapted from National Center for Health Statistics (2015). *Health, United States, 2014: With special feature on adults aged 55–64*. http://www.cdc.gov/nchs/data/hus/hus14.pdf#059, Retrieved March 21, 2016.

**Table 6** Percentage of US Individuals With Grade 1 Obesity (BMI 30.0–34.9), by Race/Ethnicity, 1988–2012

| | 1988–1994 | 1999–2002 | 2002–2006 | 2009–2012 |
|---|---|---|---|---|
| Non-Hispanic White female | 13.1 | 16.6 | 17.3 | 17.3 |
| Black or African-American female | 18.7 | 21.7 | 23.5 | 27.6 |

Adapted from National Center for Health Statistics (2015). *Health, United States, 2014: With special feature on adults aged 55–64.* http://www.cdc.gov/nchs/data/hus/hus14.pdf#059, Retrieved March 21, 2016.

**Table 7** Percentage of US Individuals With Grade 2 Obesity (BMI 35.0–39.9), by Race/Ethnicity, 1988–2012

| | 1988–1994 | 1999–2002 | 2002–2006 | 2009–2012 |
|---|---|---|---|---|
| Non-Hispanic White female | 6.2 | 9.1 | 8.5 | 8.9 |
| Black or African-American female | 10.4 | 13.5 | 15.3 | 12.9 |

Adapted from National Center for Health Statistics (2015). *Health, United States, 2014: With special feature on adults aged 55–64.* http://www.cdc.gov/nchs/data/hus/hus14.pdf#059, Retrieved March 21, 2016.

**Table 8** Percentage of US Individuals With Grade 3 Obesity (BMI $\geq$40.0), by Race/Ethnicity, 1988–2012

| | 1988–1994 | 1999–2002 | 2002–2006 | 2009–2012 |
|---|---|---|---|---|
| Non-Hispanic White female | 3.5 | 5.5 | 6.3 | 7.2 |
| Black or African-American female | 8.0 | 13.4 | 14.2 | 16.9 |

Adapted from National Center for Health Statistics (2015). *Health, United States, 2014: With special feature on adults aged 55–64.* http://www.cdc.gov/nchs/data/hus/hus14.pdf#059, Retrieved March 21, 2016.

## 2.6 Disparities in Overweight/Obesity and Physical Activity in Breast Cancer Survivors

Data show a rising trend in the United States toward significantly increased prevalence rates of obesity among women ages 60 years and older between 2011 and 2012 (from 31.5% to 38.1%; $p = 0.006$) (Ogden et al., 2014). Obesity is highly prevalent among BCa survivors (Fazzino, Sporn, & Befort, 2016; Paxton et al., 2010). This is a major public health problem because overweight and obesity are significant risk factors for recurrence (Fazzino et al., 2016; Kroenke, Chen, Rosner, & Holmes, 2005), BCa-specific mortality (Chan et al., 2014; Fazzino et al., 2016), and overall mortality (Chan et al., 2014; Fazzino et al., 2016; Protani, Coory, & Martin, 2010). AA BCa survivors are 70% more likely to be obese than are EA BCa survivors (Ogden, Carroll, Kit, & Flegal, 2012; Sheppard et al., 2016).

In a study, examining the associations between physical activity, BMI, and health-related quality of life in a multiracial/ethnic sample of BCa survivors, Paxton et al. (2010) discovered that compared to women from all other racial/ethnic groups, AA women were least likely to meet minimum guidelines for physical activity and were most likely to be obese ($p < 0.05$).

Barriers to physical activity among AA BCa survivors were recently outlined by Oyekanmi and Raheem (2014). These barriers included lack of energy, lack of time, lack of facilities or space, and lack of knowledge about how to exercise, and significantly increased the risk of not meeting current physical activity guidelines. Interestingly, the study participants who were obese and less educated reported the highest number of barriers to physical activity.

## 2.7 Evidence-Based Breast Cancer Survivorship Guidelines Related to Physical Activity and Weight Management

The Centers for Disease Control and Prevention recommend that adults in the general population engage in a minimum of 30 min of moderate-intensity physical activity for at least 5 days per week, or at least 20 min of vigorous-intensity activity for at least 3 days per week (Centers for Disease Control (CDC), 2008). Moderate-intensity physical activity is defined as aerobic exercise that raises a person's heart rate and causes them to sweat. Typically, people exercising at this level of intensity can talk but cannot sing the words to a song. In contrast, vigorous-intensity aerobic exercise occurs when a person is breathing hard and their heart rate has significantly increased. A person working out at this level of intensity is unable to say more than a few words without having to stop to breathe.

For BCa survivors, the National Comprehensive Cancer Network, Inc. (NCCN) relies on these published CDC physical activity guidelines, suggesting that survivors who follow the guidelines could reap benefits such as reducing the chance of BCa recurrence. The NCCN guidelines (National Comprehensive Cancer Network, 2016) also note that exercise reduces the number of excess fat cells in the body that produce the high levels of estrogen that are associated with BCa, and could potentially inhibit other hormones that may play a key role in BCa development.

The American Cancer Society recommends that to prevent cancer (and perhaps to prevent cancer recurrence as well), adults engage in at least 150 min of moderate-intensity physical activity per week, or at least 75 min of vigorous-intensity physical activity per week (American Cancer Society, 2016b).

# 3. CONCLUSIONS AND FUTURE DIRECTIONS

## 3.1 Multilevel Intervention Approach to Reduce Obesity (Thereby Reducing Breast Cancer Risk)

Dietary choices and physical activity are modifiable via multilevel intervention approaches addressing behavioral and environmental contributors to obesity/overweight. The obesity epidemic in the United States is largely due to an obesogenic environment in which overeating and sedentary lifestyles play a major role. An "obesogenic" environment refers to the "surroundings, opportunities, or conditions of life…that promote obesity in individuals or populations" (Swinburn, Egger, & Raza, 1999).

A limitation of many prior weight-reduction interventions is their focus on individuals rather than on both the individual and the environmental context in which he or she lives. If individuals successfully achieve weight loss but live in neighborhoods that lack a strong focus on physical activity and attend churches that serve weekly fat-laden dinners, their ability to maintain their weight loss will be severely undermined. This is the case with many past interventions.

## 3.2 The Social Ecological Model Provides a Basis for Interventions with Multilevel Approaches to Reducing Obesity/Overweight

The social ecological model (SEM) provides a multilevel framework for developing interventions to reduce obesity/overweight in BCa survivors (Bronfenbrenner, 1977; Fleury & Lee, 2006; McLeroy, Bibeau, Steckler, & Glanz, 1998). In the SEM, the multiple effects of multiple levels of influence in an environment are hypothesized to interact to influence obesity/overweight outcomes. The SEM postulates that an individual's behavior, such as losing weight and maintaining weight loss, is impacted by and impacts factors on several levels of influence. To successfully maintain weight loss, it is necessary to modify multiple aspects of the environment to support behavior change. The cumulative effects of a comprehensive approach that include simultaneously modifying intrapersonal factors, interpersonal factors, and other factors such as organizational relationships, and community/institutional policies will produce more robust and longer-term weight management outcomes than would be produced by merely focusing on the individual in isolation from his or her environmental context (Gregson et al., 2001).

As noted, behavioral interventions that target multiple levels of environmental influence are likely to produce the strongest results in achieving and maintaining weight loss among intervention participants. Multilevel interventions are defined as those that address at least two levels of influence, such as interpersonal and community/institution factors (Taplin et al., 2012). The multiple levels of influence that may influence eating and exercise habits include:

- Intrapersonal factors related to weight loss/weight loss maintenance
  - Preferences for weight loss
  - Perceptions of their body image as healthy or unhealthy
  - Knowledge about how to achieve and maintain a healthy weight
  - Skills in doing so
  - Self-confidence
  - Motivation to achieve and maintain a healthy weight
  - Sociodemographic characteristics that impact their ability to lose weight and keep it off, such as their age, SES, and health status (including comorbidities)
- Interpersonal relationships related to weight loss/weight loss maintenance
  - Family, friends, and social networks
  - Culture
  - Food availability at home
  - Social support
  - Time constraints to prepare food
- Community/institutional factors related to weight loss/weight loss maintenance
  - Food availability at stores
  - Socioeconomic characteristics of the community
  - Options for eating out, portion sizes at restaurants, and the built environment (safe walking trails, etc.)
  - Access to healthy, nourishing food at reasonable prices
- Macrolevel/public policy related to weight loss/weight loss maintenance
  - Media—which types of food are widely advertised in the local community (unhealthy vs healthy food choices)

- Public policy regarding neighborhood safety to promote participation in outdoor activities
- Development/zoning regulations and the availability of parks and other forms of outdoor recreation
- The price of food at local stores.

The SEM helps to identify opportunities for weight loss and management interventions by demonstrating how the multiple levels of influence impact weight-related outcomes. For example, at the policy level, employers could have reduced employee-borne health insurance coverage costs for those at a healthy weight. At the institutional level, interventions could focus on employer policies that promoted walking programs at work. At the community level, interventions could focus on improved pedestrian safety. At the interpersonal level, interventions could focus on weight management and physical activity interventions at the group level, with family, work colleagues, or peers such as church members rather than at the individual level. On each of these levels, social change theories that could be employed to promote weight loss/weight loss maintenance include Social Cognitive Theory (which examines the dynamic ways in which personal factors and environmental factors influence each other), Community Organization and Community Based Participatory Models (which focus on community-led approaches to evaluating and reducing the prevalence of obesity/overweight), Diffusion of Innovations Theory (which demonstrates how new social practices spread within an organization, community or society), and Communication Theory (which demonstrates how different means of communication produce different health outcomes) (Washington State Department of Health, 2012).

Finally, on the intrapersonal level, interventions could employ cognitive behavioral change theories such as the Health Belief Model (which focuses on perception of a threat to health such as obesity, the health benefits of losing weight, and the factors that impact the decision to lose weight) (Stretcher & Rosenstock, 1997), the Stages of Change (Transtheoretical) Model (which evaluates motivation and readiness to engage in health behavior such as weight loss) (Prochaska & DiClemente, 1983), or the Theory of Planned Behavior (Ajzen, 1991) to help promote weight management (which evaluates the interactions among beliefs, attitudes, intentions, behavior, and perceived control over behavior such as weight loss activities). According to the Theory of Planned Behavior, intention to engage in healthy behavior is the most significant predictor of actually engaging in the behavior.

Recently, Fazzino et al. (2016) developed and tested a 6-month group phone-based weight loss intervention for rural BCa survivors. The intervention included elements of the SEM by focusing on a group-based design, as well as Communication Theory by disseminating the intervention via a weekly 1-h group teleconference. The intervention targeted weight loss as well as physical activity. In terms of weight loss, the participants were instructed to employ a planned meal format that included two whey-based protein shakes per day, two portion-controlled factory-frozen meals per day, and a minimum of five fruits or vegetables per day. The American College of Sports Medicine's physical activity guidelines of completing 225 min/week of moderate-intensity physical activity were used as the culminating physical activity goal, with activity gradually increased per week to meet this goal. Most of the participants chose brisk walking as their preferred form of exercise. During the teleconferences, common barriers to healthy eating and physical activity were discussed and problem solving was used to overcome the barriers. During each weekly call, each participant reported to the group whether they had met their dietary and physical activity goals for the week. Of the 186 rural, obese BCa survivors ($\geq$3 months from initial cancer treatment; BMI 27–45, with physician clearance) who participated in the intervention, clinically meaningful weight loss (>5%) was reported in 91% of the participants. Weight loss was confirmed via morning fasting weigh-in assessments at baseline, and at 6-, 12-, 18-, and 24-month postrandomization (Fazzino et al., 2016). Height was measured at baseline with a stadiometer, and waist circumference was obtained with two measurements per site within 2 cm (Befort et al., 2014).

## 3.3 Relevance of the SEM for Obesity Reduction Interventions with AA Women Who Are Breast Cancer Survivors

The SEM has particular relevance for efforts to reduce obesity and overweight among AA women. As Kumanyika et al. (2007) point out, the causes of obesity among AA women are related to core social environmental factors and therefore interventions to reduce obesity in this population must address these factors. For example, a recent study shows that financial and work-related stress were significant contributors to high levels of obesity among AA women, suggesting that employee health programs could consider the issue of job strain and its impact on the health of employees, and implement employee health programs to decrease stress, reduce obesity, and improve employee health outcomes (Moore-Greene et al., 2012). Race and ethnicity influence life contexts and impact factors that relate to eating and physical activity behaviors (Kumanyika et al., 2007).

SEM approaches that take into account cultural and contextual factors of AA communities are more likely than other approaches to achieve success in obesity/overweight-reduction interventions. For example, a SEM approach to obesity reduction in AA populations was developed by Kumanyika et al. (2007). Their approach focuses on four themes related to the inclusion of community and family life contexts in obesity research. These themes include community-specific environmental influences, community structure and organization, women as a central focus, and heterogeneity in the AA population. Community-specific environmental influences include poor housing, financial constraints on food choices and lack of availability of recreational activities. Community structure and organization refer to formal and informal social networks and sources of social support. Women as a central focus refer to the influential roles many AA women play as the heads of their households. Heterogeneity refers to the fact, as has been pointed out, that there is considerable within-group diversity among AA women in terms of SES as well as neighborhood characteristics, urban vs rural differences, and religion. An important point that is made by these authors is the need to provide direct economic benefits to the communities that participate in obesity reduction efforts.

SEM approaches for obesity/overweight reduction could also address the issue of collectivism, which is a more prevalent value among AAs than among members of many other groups (Gilbert, Harvey, & Belgrave, 2009). Collectivism refers to a belief that the basic element of society is the family rather than the individual (Steele-Moses et al., 2009). In a recent review, Kuo identified the prominence of collective coping behaviors among African Americans and Asian Americans (Kuo, 2013). Religiosity, another prevalent value among AAs, could also be addressed in SEM approaches. Religiosity refers to a range of activities including church attendance, prayer, and belief in God as a causal agent (Kreuter et al., 2005). In a randomized trial with 1227 lower-income AA women from 10 urban public health centers, Kreuter et al. (2005) found that women who received behavioral construct (BCT, consisting of individualized approaches that do not take contextual variables into account) tailoring plus culturally relevant tailoring (focusing on religiosity, collectivism, racial pride, and present time orientation) produced significantly higher rates of receipt of mammography and increases in daily consumption of fruits and vegetables compared with women who received BCT alone, CRT alone, or the control group. Racial pride refers to interest and involvement in traditional AA cultural practices such as serving collard greens and black-eyed peas on New Year's Day for good luck. Time orientation reflects a tendency to think and act based on immediate, rather than more distal, consequences, perhaps due to the issue of coping with daily stressors (Lukwago, Kreuter, Bucholtz, Holt, & Clark, 2001). Interestingly, instruments to measure collectivism, religiosity, racial pride, and time orientation among AA women have been previously developed and validated (Lukwago et al., 2001).

To cite an example of how an intervention could be developed to promote weight loss in AA women, the results of a study by James et al. (2012) could be extended to intervention development. They conducted a study in which they used the Health Belief Model to develop culturally appropriate weight management materials in a study with 50 AA women. Their findings show that perceived benefits of weight loss included reduced risk for health problems, improved physical appearance, and improved quality of life. Perceived barriers included lack of motivation, lack of trustworthy nutrition information, and social support. Motivators to weight loss included diagnosis of a health problem, physical appearance, and saving money on clothes. These findings could be used to develop an intervention that included multiple levels of influence such as employing social support to aid women in their weight loss goals, community interventions to enhance opportunities for physical activity, making reliable nutrition information readily available in local grocery stores, and working with local clothiers to offer price reductions to women who could demonstrate weight loss over a specified period of time. Interventions could also address targeted marketing of high-calorie foods and beverages in AA communities (Grier & Kumanyika, 2008).

More recently, Sheppard et al. (2016) conducted a diet and exercise trial with overweight and obese AA BCa survivors. This two-arm randomized trial tested the effectiveness of a culturally targeted 12-week lifestyle intervention ($n=16$) vs usual care ($n=15$). The intervention was developed with input from survivors who were representative of the end-users. The intervention included content related to faith and spirituality, foods that are relevant to AAs, and body image perceptions (Sheppard et al., 2016). Additionally, the risk information that was presented to the intervention group participants included information that was pertinent to AA cancer survivors. The intervention, titled "Stepping STONE (Survivors Taking on Nutrition and Exercise)," was offered to AA BCa survivors who were between 6 months and 5 years postactive treatment, and who were overweight or obese (BMI $\geq 25$ kg/m$^2$ or BMI $\leq 40$ kg/m$^2$, respectively; thus excluding morbidly obese survivors) and were survivors of early stage/localized BCa. The Stepping STONE intervention incorporated elements of the Theory of Planned Behavior and Social Cognitive Theory and individualized sessions were tailored to participant's intentions, attitudes, and subjective norms toward dietary changes and physical activity that were expressed at baseline. Importantly and highly relevant to the SEM, the intervention includes actionable steps, such as empowering participants to include their families in identifying and preparing healthier meal options (Sheppard et al., 2016). Thus, by developing strategies to influence participants' social networks, environmental influences on behavior were addressed. Other such influences included barriers to exercise, in which strategies were identified to foster participant's engagement in physical activity within the constraints of their neighborhoods/towns. The physical activity recommendations in the Stepping STONE intervention included moderate-intensity exercise for at least 30 min per day for 5 or more days per week, and the dietary recommendations included consuming at least five fruits and vegetables per day, with less than 35% of daily calories from total fat. The results of the Stepping STONE intervention showed that the intervention group did not meet the 5% weight loss target, instead losing only 0.8%. However, BMI improved and physical activity levels were higher in the intervention group than in the usual care group.

In summary, few studies demonstrate how to effectively conduct obesity reduction and weight management interventions with AA women (Kumanyika et al., 2011). However, recent multisite efficacy trials of lifestyle interventions (using an intervention adapted from the Diabetes Prevention Program that includes group sessions with registered dietitians, behavioral psychologists, and exercise specialists) to reduce obesity have shown clinically significant weight reductions for AA and Hispanic adults (Wadden et al., 2009). More studies are greatly needed to translate these efficacy findings into community-based interventions given the looming health crisis among AA women.

## ACKNOWLEDGMENTS

The authors wish to acknowledge the following funding sources: South Carolina Cancer Disparities Research Center (SC CaDRe; P20 CA157071); Medical University of South Carolina—Cancer Center Support Grant (P30 CA138313); Improving Resection Rates among African Americans with NSCLC (R01 MD005892); and Getting Onboard with an Active Lifestyle to Reduce the Risk of Breast Cancer Recurrence (G.O.A.L. Study) (Hollings Cancer Center CTO: 101942).

## REFERENCES

Ajzen, I. (1991). The theory of planned behavior. *Organizational Behavior and Human Decision Processes*, *50*, 179–211.

American Cancer Society. (2008). *Cancer facts and figures*. Atlanta, GA: American Cancer Society, Inc., Surveillance Health Policy Research.

American Cancer Society. (2016a). *Cancer facts & figures for African Americans 2016–2018*. Atlanta, GA: American Cancer Society.

American Cancer Society. (2016b). *American Cancer Society Guidelines on nutrition and physical activity for cancer prevention*. Atlanta, GA: American Cancer Society.

Bach, P. B., Schrag, D., Brawley, O. W., Galaznik, A., Yakren, S., & Begg, C. B. (2002). Survival of blacks and whites after a cancer diagnosis. *JAMA*, *287*(16), 2106–2113.

Barnes, A. S., & Kimbro, R. T. (2012). Descriptive study of educated African American women successful at weight-loss maintenance through lifestyle changes. *Journal of General Internal Medicine*, *27*(10), 1272–1279. http://dx.doi.org/10.1007/s11606-012-2060-2.

Befort, C. A., Klemp, J. R., Fabian, C., Perri, M. G., Sullivan, D. K., Schmitz, K. H., … Shireman, T. (2014). Protocol and recruitment results from a randomized controlled trial comparing group phone-based versus newsletter interventions for weight loss maintenance among rural breast cancer survivors. *Contemporary Clinical Trials*, *37*(2), 261–271. http://dx.doi.org/10.1016/j.cct.2014.01.010.

Bronfenbrenner, U. (1977). Toward an experimental ecology of human development. *American Psychologist*, *32*, 513–531.

Brown, K. A., & Simpson, E. R. (2012). Obesity and breast cancer: Mechanisms and therapeutic implications. *Frontiers in Bioscience (Elite Edition)*, *4*, 2515–2524.

Campbell, K. L., Foster-Schubert, K. E., Alfano, C. M., Wang, C. C., Wang, C. Y., Duggan, C. R., … McTiernan, A. (2012). Reduced-calorie dietary weight loss, exercise, and sex hormones in postmenopausal women: Randomized controlled trial. *Journal of Clinical Oncology*, *30*(19), 2314–2326. http://dx.doi.org/10.1200/JCO.2011.37.9792.

Campbell, K. L., Van Patten, C. L., Neil, S. E., Kirkham, A. A., Gotay, C. C., Gelmon, K. A., & McKenzie, D. C. (2012). Feasibility of a lifestyle intervention on body weight and serum biomarkers in breast cancer survivors with overweight and obesity. *Journal of the Academy of Nutrition and Dietetics*, *112*(4), 559–567. http://dx.doi.org/10.1016/j.jada.2011.10.022.

Cecchini, R. S., Costantino, J. P., Cauley, J. A., Cronin, W. M., Wickerham, D. L., Land, S. R., … Wolmark, N. (2012). Body mass index and the risk for developing invasive breast cancer among high-risk women in NSABP P-1 and STAR breast cancer prevention trials. *Cancer Prevention Research (Philadelphia, PA)*, *5*(4), 583–592. http://dx.doi.org/10.1158/1940-6207.CAPR-11-0482.

Centers for Disease Control (CDC). (2008). *Physical activity guidelines for Americans*. Atlanta, GA: Centers for Disease Control and Prevention.

Centers for Disease Control and Prevention (CDC) (2015). Behavioral risk factor surveillance system. *Prevalence of self-reported obesity among U.S. adults by state and territory, BRFSS, 2015*. Retrieved from, https://www.cdc.gov/obesity/data/prevalence-maps.html.

Centers for Disease Control and Prevention. (2016). *FastStats on obesity and overweight*. Atlanta, GA: Centers for Disease Control and Prevention. Retrieved March 21, from, http://www.cdc.gov/nchs/fastats/obesity-overweight.htm.

Chan, D. S., Vieira, A. R., Aune, D., Bandera, E. V., Greenwood, D. C., McTiernan, A., … Norat, T. (2014). Body mass index and survival in women with breast cancer-systematic literature review and meta-analysis of 82 follow-up studies. *Annals of Oncology*, *25*(10), 1901–1914. http://dx.doi.org/10.1093/annonc/mdu042.

Clarke, P., O'Malley, P. M., Johnston, L. D., & Schulenberg, J. E. (2009). Social disparities in BMI trajectories across adulthood by gender, race/ethnicity and lifetime socio-economic

position: 1986–2004. *International Journal of Epidemiology, 38*(2), 499–509. http://dx.doi.org/10.1093/ije/dyn214.
Coogan, P. E., Wise, L. A., Cozier, Y. C., Palmer, J. R., & Rosenberg, L. (2012). Lifecourse educational status in relation to weight gain in African American women. *Ethnicity & Disease, 22*(2), 198–206.
Costa, C., Incio, J., & Soares, R. (2007). Angiogenesis and chronic inflammation: Cause or consequence? *Angiogenesis, 10*(3), 149–166. http://dx.doi.org/10.1007/s10456-007-9074-0.
Daly, B., & Olopade, O. I. (2015). A perfect storm: How tumor biology, genomics, and health care delivery patterns collide to create a racial survival disparity in breast cancer and proposed interventions for change. *CA: A Cancer Journal for Clinicians, 65*(3), 221–238. http://dx.doi.org/10.3322/caac.21271.
Danforth, D. N., Jr. (2013). Disparities in breast cancer outcomes between Caucasian and African American women: A model for describing the relationship of biological and non-biological factors. *Breast Cancer Research, 15*(3), 208. http://dx.doi.org/10.1186/bcr3429.
D'Arcy, M., Fleming, J., Robinson, W. R., Kirk, E. L., Perou, C. M., & Troester, M. A. (2015). Race-associated biological differences among luminal a breast tumors. *Breast Cancer Research and Treatment, 152*(2), 437–448. http://dx.doi.org/10.1007/s10549-015-3474-4.
Demark-Wahnefried, W., Campbell, K. L., & Hayes, S. C. (2012). Weight management and its role in breast cancer rehabilitation. *Cancer, 118*(8 Suppl.), 2277–2287. http://dx.doi.org/10.1002/cncr.27466.
DeSantis, C. E., Siegel, R. L., Sauer, A. G., Miller, K. D., Fedewa, S. A., Alcaraz, K. I., & Jemal, A. (2016). Cancer statistics for African Americans, 2016: Progress and opportunities in reducing racial disparities. *CA: A Cancer Journal for Clinicians, 66*(4), 290–308. http://dx.doi.org/10.3322/caac.21340.
Dietze, E. C., Sistrunk, C., Miranda-Carboni, G., O'Regan, R., & Seewaldt, V. L. (2015). Triple-negative breast cancer in African-American women: Disparities versus biology. *Nature Reviews. Cancer, 15*(4), 248–254. http://dx.doi.org/10.1038/nrc3896.
Eliassen, A. H., Colditz, G. A., Rosner, B., Willett, W. C., & Hankinson, S. E. (2006). Adult weight change and risk of postmenopausal breast cancer. *JAMA, 296*(2), 193–201. http://dx.doi.org/10.1001/jama.296.2.193.
Fabian, C. J. (2012). Simplifying the energy balance message for breast cancer prevention. *Cancer Prevention Research (Philadelphia, PA), 5*(4), 511–514. http://dx.doi.org/10.1158/1940-6207.CAPR-12-0088.
Fazzino, T. L., Sporn, N. J., & Befort, C. A. (2016). A qualitative evaluation of a group phone-based weight loss intervention for rural breast cancer survivors: Themes and mechanisms of success. *Support Care Cancer, 24*(7), 3165–3173. http://dx.doi.org/10.1007/s00520-016-3149-7.
Fleury, J., & Lee, S. M. (2006). The social ecological model and physical activity in African American women. *American Journal of Community Psychology, 37*(1–2), 129–140. http://dx.doi.org/10.1007/s10464-005-9002-7.
Gaillard, T. R., Schuster, D., & Osei, K. (2012). Characterization of metabolically unhealthy overweight/obese African American women: Significance of insulin-sensitive and insulin-resistant phenotypes. *Journal of the National Medical Association, 104*(3–4), 164–171.
Gilbert, D. J., Harvey, A. R., & Belgrave, F. Z. (2009). Advancing the Africentric paradigm shift discourse: Building toward evidence-based Africentric interventions in social work practice with African Americans. *Social Work, 54*(3), 243–252.
Gregson, J., Foerster, S. B., Orr, R., Jones, L., Benedict, J., Clarke, B., … Zotz, A. K. (2001). System, environmental, and policy changes: Using the social-ecological model as a

framework for evaluating nutrition education and social marketing programs with low-income audiences. *Journal of Nutrition Education, 33*(Suppl. 1), S4–S15.
Grier, S. A., & Kumanyika, S. K. (2008). The context for choice: Health implications of targeted food and beverage marketing to African Americans. *American Journal of Public Health, 98*(9), 1616–1629. http://dx.doi.org/10.2105/AJPH.2007.115626.
Hoffman, H. J., Lavendra, N. L., Levine, P. H., Young, H. A., Alexander, L. M., Patierno, S. R., & District of Columbia Citywide Patient Navigator Research Program Research Group (2011). Having health insurance does not eliminate race/ethnicity-associated delays in breast cancer diagnosis in the District of Columbia. *Cancer, 117*, 3824–3832.
James, D. C., Pobee, J. W., Oxidine, D., Brown, L., & Joshi, G. (2012). Using the health belief model to develop culturally appropriate weight-management materials for African-American women. *Journal of the Academy of Nutrition and Dietetics, 112*, 664–670.
Khan, L. K., Sobush, K., Keener, D., Goodman, K., Lowry, A., Kakietek, J., & Zaro, S. (2009). Recommended community strategies and measurements to prevent obesity in the United States. *MMWR—Recommendations and Reports, 58*(RR-7), 1–26.
Komenaka, I. K., Martinez, M. E., Pennington, R. E., Jr., Hsu, C. H., Clare, S. E., Thompson, P. A., … Goulet, R. J., Jr. (2010). Race and ethnicity and breast cancer outcomes in an underinsured population. *Journal of the National Cancer Institute, 102*(15), 1178–1187. http://dx.doi.org/10.1093/jnci/djq215.
Kreuter, M. W., Sugg-Skinner, C., Holt, C. L., Clark, E. M., Haire-Joshu, D., Fu, Q., … Bucholtz, D. (2005). Cultural tailoring for mammography and fruit and vegetable intake among low-income African-American women in urban public health centers. *Preventive Medicine, 41*(1), 53–62. http://dx.doi.org/10.1016/j.ypmed.2004.10.013.
Kroenke, C. H., Chen, W. Y., Rosner, B., & Holmes, M. D. (2005). Weight, weight gain, and survival after breast cancer diagnosis. *Journal of Clinical Oncology, 23*(7), 1370–1378. http://dx.doi.org/10.1200/JCO.2005.01.079.
Kumanyika, S., Fassbender, J., Phipps, E., Tan-Torres, S., Localio, R., Morales, K. H., … Wadden, T. A. (2011). Design, recruitment and start up of a primary care weight loss trial targeting African American and Hispanic adults. *Contemporary Clinical Trials, 32*(2), 215–224. http://dx.doi.org/10.1016/j.cct.2010.11.002.
Kumanyika, S. K., Whitt-Glover, M. C., Gary, T. L., Prewitt, T. E., Odoms-Young, A. M., Banks-Wallace, J., … Samuel-Hodge, C. D. (2007). Expanding the obesity research paradigm to reach African American communities. *Preventing Chronic Disease, 4*(4), A112.
Kuo, B. C. (2013). Collectivism and coping: Current theories, evidence, and measurements of collective coping. *International Journal of Psychology, 48*(3), 374–388. http://dx.doi.org/10.1080/00207594.2011.640681.
Lahmann, P. H., Hoffmann, K., Allen, N., van Gils, C. H., Khaw, K. T., Tehard, B., … Riboli, E. (2004). Body size and breast cancer risk: Findings from the European prospective investigation into cancer and nutrition (EPIC). *International Journal of Cancer, 111*(5), 762–771. http://dx.doi.org/10.1002/ijc.20315.
Lukwago, S. N., Kreuter, M. W., Bucholtz, D. C., Holt, C. L., & Clark, E. M. (2001). Development and validation of brief scales to measure collectivism, religiosity, racial pride, and time orientation in urban African American women. *Family & Community Health, 24*(3), 63–71.
Ma, H., Lu, Y., Malone, K. E., Marchbanks, P. A., Deapen, D. M., Spirtas, R., … Bernstein, L. (2013). Mortality risk of black women and white women with invasive breast cancer by hormone receptors, HER2, and p53 status. *BMC Cancer, 13*, 225. http://dx.doi.org/10.1186/1471-2407-13-225.
Mack, K. A., Anderson, L., Galuska, D., Zablotsky, D., Holtzman, D., & Ahluwalia, I. (2004). Health and sociodemographic factors associated with body weight and weight

objectives for women: 2000 behavioral risk factor surveillance system. *Journal of Women's Health (2002)*, *13*(9), 1019–1032. http://dx.doi.org/10.1089/jwh.2004.13.1019.

McCarthy, A. M., Yang, J., & Armstrong, K. (2015). Increasing disparities in breast cancer mortality from 1979 to 2010 for US black women aged 20 to 49 years. *American Journal of Public Health*, *105*(Suppl. 3), S446–S448. http://dx.doi.org/10.2105/AJPH.2014.302297.

McLeroy, K. R., Bibeau, D., Steckler, A., & Glanz, K. (1988). An ecological perspective on health promotion programs. *Health Education Quarterly*, *15*(4), 351–377.

Moore-Greene, G. M., Gross, S. M., Silver, K. D., & Perrino, C. S. (2012). Chronic stress and decreased physical exercise: Impact on weight for African American women. *Ethnicity & Disease*, *22*(2), 185–191.

Morimoto, L. M., White, E., Chen, Z., Chlebowski, R. T., Hays, J., Kuller, L., … McTiernan, A. (2002). Obesity, body size, and risk of postmenopausal breast cancer: The women's health initiative (United States). *Cancer Causes & Control*, *13*(8), 741–751.

National Center for Health Statistics (2015). *Health, United States, 2014: With Special feature on adults aged 55–64*. Hyattsville, MD.

National Comprehensive Cancer Network (2016). *Exercise for life [patient and caregiver resources]*. National Comprehensive Cancer Network, Inc. (NCCN). Retrieved from, https://www.nccn.org/patients/resources/life_after_cancer/exercise.aspx.

Ogden, C. L., Carroll, M. D., Curtin, L. R., McDowell, M. A., Tabak, C. J., & Flegal, K. M. (2006). Prevalence of overweight and obesity in the United States, 1999–2004. *JAMA*, *295*(13), 1549–1555. http://dx.doi.org/10.1001/jama.295.13.1549.

Ogden, C. L., Carroll, M. D., Kit, B. K., & Flegal, K. M. (2012). Prevalence of obesity in the United States, 2009–2010. *NCHS Data Brief*, *82*, 1–8.

Ogden, C. L., Carroll, M. D., Kit, B. K., & Flegal, K. M. (2014). Prevalence of childhood and adult obesity in the United States, 2011–2012. *JAMA*, *311*(8), 806–814. http://dx.doi.org/10.1001/jama.2014.732.

Oyekanmi, G., & Raheem, P. (2014). Barriers to physical activity among African American breast cancer survivors. *Psychooncology*, *14*(23), 1314–1317.

Palmer, J. R., Viscidi, E., Troester, M. A., Hong, C. C., Schedin, P., Bethea, T. N., … Ambrosone, C. B. (2014). Parity, lactation, and breast cancer subtypes in African American women: Results from the AMBER consortium. *Journal of the National Cancer Institute*, *106*(10). http://dx.doi.org/10.1093/jnci/dju237.

Paxton, R. J., Phillips, K. L., Jones, L. A., Chang, S., Taylor, W. C., Courneya, K. S., & Pierce, J. P. (2010). Associations among physical activity, body mass index, and health-related quality of life by race/ethnicity in a diverse sample of breast cancer survivors. *Cancer*, *118*, 4024–4031.

Phipps, A. I., Chlebowski, R. T., Prentice, R., McTiernan, A., Wactawski-Wende, J., Kuller, L. H., … Li, C. I. (2011). Reproductive history and oral contraceptive use in relation to risk of triple-negative breast cancer. *Journal of the National Cancer Institute*, *103*(6), 470–477. http://dx.doi.org/10.1093/jnci/djr030.

Pischon, T., Nothlings, U., & Boeing, H. (2008). Obesity and cancer. *The Proceedings of the Nutrition Society*, *67*(2), 128–145. http://dx.doi.org/10.1017/S0029665108006976.

Pizot, C., Boniol, M., Mullie, P., Koechlin, A., Boniol, M., Boyle, P., & Autier, P. (2016). Physical activity, hormone replacement therapy and breast cancer risk: A meta-analysis of prospective studies. *European Journal of Cancer*, *52*, 138–154. http://dx.doi.org/10.1016/j.ejca.2015.10.063.

Press, R., Carrasquillo, O., Sciacca, R. R., & Giardina, E. G. (2008). Racial/ethnic disparities in time to follow-up after an abnormal mammogram. *Journal of Women's Health (2002)*, *17*(6), 923–930. http://dx.doi.org/10.1089/jwh.2007.0402.

Prochaska, J. O., & DiClemente, C. C. (1983). Stages and processes of self-change of smoking: Toward an integrative model of change. *Journal of Consulting and Clinical Psychology, 51*(3), 390–395.

Protani, M., Coory, M., & Martin, J. H. (2010). Effect of obesity on survival of women with breast cancer: Systematic review and meta-analysis. *Breast Cancer Research and Treatment, 123*(3), 627–635. http://dx.doi.org/10.1007/s10549-010-0990-0.

Reeder-Hayes, K. E., Wheeler, S. B., & Mayer, D. K. (2015). Health disparities across the breast cancer continuum. *Seminars in Oncology Nursing, 31*(2), 170–177. http://dx.doi.org/10.1016/j.soncn.2015.02.005.

Renehan, A. G., Roberts, D. L., & Dive, C. (2008). Obesity and cancer: Pathophysiological and biological mechanisms. *Archives of Physiology and Biochemistry, 114*(1), 71–83. http://dx.doi.org/10.1080/13813450801954303.

Sauaia, A., & Byers, T. (2012). Obesity in US children and adults. *JAMA, 307*(20), 2145. http://dx.doi.org/10.1001/jama.2012.4726 author reply 2145–2146.

Sheppard, V. B., Hicks, J., Makambi, K., Hurtado-de-Mendoza, A., Demark-Wahnefried, W., & Adams-Campbell, L. (2016). The feasibility and acceptability of a diet and exercise trial in overweight and obese black breast cancer survivors: The stepping STONE study. *Contemporary Clinical Trials, 46*, 106–113. http://dx.doi.org/10.1016/j.cct.2015.12.005.

Smith-Bindman, R., Miqlioretti, D. L., Lurie, N., Abraham, L., Barbash, R. B., Strzelczyk, J., … Kerlikowske, K. (2006). Does utilization of screening mammography explain racial and ethnic differences in breast cancer? *Annals of Internal Medicine, 144*, 541–553.

Steele-Moses, S. K., Russell, K. M., Kreuter, M., Monahan, P., Bourff, S., & Champion, V. L. (2009). Cultural constructs, stage of change, and adherence to mammography among low-income African American women. *Journal of Health Care for the Poor and Underserved, 20*(1), 257–273. http://dx.doi.org/10.1353/hpu.0.0123.

Stretcher, V. J., & Rosenstock, I. (1997). The health belief model. In F. M. L.ewis, K. Glanz, & B. Rimer (Eds.), *Health behavior and health education: Theory, research and practice,* (2nd ed.), San Francisco, CA: Jossey-Bass Inc. (pp. 41–59).

Swinburn, B., Egger, G., & Raza, F. (1999). Dissecting obesogenic environments: The development and application of a framework for identifying and prioritizing environmental interventions for obesity. *Preventive Medicine, 29*(6 Pt 1), 563–570. http://dx.doi.org/10.1006/pmed.1999.0585.

Tao, L., Gomez, S. L., Keegan, T. H., Kurian, A. W., & Clarke, C. A. (2015). Breast cancer mortality in African-American and non-hispanic white women by molecular subtype and stage at diagnosis: A population-based study. *Cancer Epidemiology, Biomarkers & Prevention, 24*(7), 1039–1045. http://dx.doi.org/10.1158/1055-9965.EPI-15-0243.

Taplin, S. H., Anhang Price, R., Edwards, H. M., Foster, M. K., Breslau, E. S., Chollette, V., … Zapka, J. (2012). Introduction: Understanding and influencing multilevel factors across the cancer care continuum. *Journal of the National Cancer Institute Monographs, 2012*(44), 2–10. http://dx.doi.org/10.1093/jncimonographs/lgs008.

Wadden, T. A., West, D. S., Neiberg, R. H., Wing, R. R., Ryan, D. H., Johnson, K. C., … Look, A. R. G. (2009). One-year weight losses in the look AHEAD study: Factors associated with success. *Obesity (Silver Spring), 17*(4), 713–722. http://dx.doi.org/10.1038/oby.2008.637.

Wang, Y., & Chen, X. (2011). How much of racial/ethnic disparities in dietary intakes, exercise, and weight status can be explained by nutrition and health-related psychosocial factors and socioeconomic status among US adults? *Journal of American Dietetic Association, 111*, 1904–1911.

Wang, Y., & Chen, X. (2012). Between-group differences in nutrition and health-related psychosocial factors among US adults and their associations with diet, exercise, and weight status. *Journal of Academy of Nutrition and Dietetics*, *112*. 486–498 e483.

Warner, E. T., Tamimi, R. M., Hughes, M. E., Ottesen, R. A., Wong, Y. N., Edge, S. B., … Partridge, A. H. (2015). Racial and ethnic differences in breast cancer survival: Mediating effect of tumor characteristics and sociodemographic and treatment factors. *Journal of Clinical Oncology*, *33*(20), 2254–2261. http://dx.doi.org/10.1200/JCO.2014.57.1349.

Washington State Department of Health. (2012). *Partners in action: Good nutrition, active living & healthy communities*. Seattle, WA: Washington State Department of Health. UW Center for Public Health Nutrition.

Yang, X. R., Sherman, M. E., Rimm, D. L., Lissowska, J., Brinton, L. A., Peplonska, B., … Garcia-Closas, M. (2007). Differences in risk factors for breast cancer molecular subtypes in a population-based study. *Cancer Epidemiology, Biomarkers & Prevention*, *16*(3), 439–443. http://dx.doi.org/10.1158/1055-9965.EPI-06-0806.

CHAPTER THREE

# MicroRNAs and Their Impact on Breast Cancer, the Tumor Microenvironment, and Disparities

**A. Evans-Knowell*, A.C. LaRue[†,‡,§], V.J. Findlay[‡,§,1]**

*South Carolina State University, Orangeburg, SC, United States
[†]Research Services, Ralph H. Johnson VAMC, Medical University of South Carolina, Charleston, SC, United States
[‡]Medical University of South Carolina, Charleston, SC, United States
[§]Hollings Cancer Center, Medical University of South Carolina, Charleston, SC, United States
[1]Corresponding author: e-mail address: findlay@musc.edu

## Contents



## Abstract

Breast cancer is a worldwide health issue as it represents the leading cause of cancer in women and the second-leading cause of cancer-related mortality in women, with an increasing incidence. Nothing speaks more clearly to the shocking breast cancer health disparities than the fact that African American (AA) women are as likely to get breast cancer as Caucasian American (CA) women, yet have a higher breast cancer death rate. It is becoming increasingly apparent that racial disparity in cancer exists due to molecular differences in tumor biology as well as, or in addition to, socioeconomic and standard of care issues (Albain, Unger, Crowley, Coltman, & Hershman, 2009). A greater

*Advances in Cancer Research*, Volume 133
ISSN 0065-230X
http://dx.doi.org/10.1016/bs.acr.2016.08.003

understanding of the risk factors and biological links associated with breast cancer, will significantly impact AA communities due to the higher deaths associated with this disease in this population. microRNAs are small noncoding RNA molecules that were recently discovered as major players in the regulation of many diseases including cancer. Although, there are many studies that have investigated the role of miRNAs in breast cancer, few have investigated their role if any in breast cancer disparities. This review serves to summarize the current published literature that is involved in the study of microRNAs and their impact on breast cancer disparities.

# 1. INTRODUCTION

## 1.1 Breast Cancer

Breast cancer is the most commonly diagnosed cancer in women. In 2016, an estimated 234,000 new cases of breast cancer are expected to be diagnosed in women in the United States (Siegel, Miller, & Jemal, 2015). Breast cancer is also the second-leading cause of death among women; in fact, this accounts for 15% of all cancer deaths (DeSantis et al., 2016). Breast cancer is clinically classified into three subtypes based on the expression of the estrogen receptor (ER), progesterone receptor (PR), and human epidermal growth factor receptor 2 (HER2) as (1) hormone receptor positive (ER+/PR+), (2) HER2+, or (3) triple negative (the absence of all three receptors) (Ali et al., 2016; Inoue & Fry, 2016). It is becoming increasingly recognized as a heterogeneous disease with multiple subtypes based on molecular profiling that was used to show that breast cancer comprises at least seven different biologic subtypes (Sorlie et al., 2001), that includes luminal A, luminal B, luminal C, HER2-enriched, basal-like, claudin-low, and normal breast-like (for a review, see Kittaneh, Montero, & Gluck, 2013).

## 1.2 Breast Cancer Disparities

It has been well established that breast cancer affects African American (AA) women at disproportionate rates, AA women now have the same incidence rates as Caucasian American (CA) women, yet they have a higher breast cancer mortality rate (American Cancer Society, 2016; DeSantis et al., 2016). According to 2016 statistics from the American Cancer Society, breast cancer leads the list with 32% for the estimated highest number of new cases (30,700) in AA women. It is expected that one in nine AA women will develop breast cancer in their lifetime, while 1 in

31 will die from the disease (DeSantis et al., 2016). Surprisingly, while the disparity gap is narrowing in colon, lung, and prostate cancer (DeSantis et al., 2016), it is continuing to widen in breast cancer (Siegel, Ward, Brawley, & Jemal, 2011; Smith et al., 2011). Advancements in cancer treatment, screening, and diagnosis are helping women overall, however breast cancer incidence and death rates in AA women are steadily increasing (Zeng et al., 2015). Currently, the 5-year relative survival rate is 80% for AA women compared to 91% among CA women (DeSantis et al., 2016). Indeed, racial disparities in cancer outcomes have been observed in several malignancies. It is believed that biological and nonbiological factors play a major role in breast cancer disparity. Nonbiological factors include socioeconomic factors, access to healthcare, cultural factors, and comorbidities. A study by the Hershman group found that, after controlling for stage, demographics, socioeconomic variables, tumor characteristics, and treatment factors, disparity remained among both premenopausal and postmenopausal women who were diagnosed with early stage breast cancer (Albain et al., 2009). Therefore, it is clear that even with considerations of nonbiological factors, breast cancer racial disparities still exist due to poorly understood inherent molecular and genetic differences in tumor biology. Therefore, a greater understanding of these biological factors is critical for addressing the increased cancer mortality observed in AA women.

## 1.3 microRNAs

microRNAs (miRNAs) are endogenous 19–25 nucleotide noncoding RNAs that have emerged as a novel class of small, evolutionary conserved gene regulatory molecules involved in key developmental and cellular functions (He & Hannon, 2004; Wiemer, 2007). They primarily regulate gene expression by acting on target mRNAs and promoting either degradation or translational repression, depending upon complementarity (Ambros, 2004; Bartel, 2004; He & Hannon, 2004). They comprise ~3% of the human genome and regulate ~30% of transcripts (Cummins & Velculescu, 2006; Kent & Mendell, 2006). Based on location, miRNAs can be grouped into two classes, intergenic and intragenic. Intergenic miRNAs are located between protein-coding genes while intragenic miRNAs are located within the introns of protein-coding genes (Yao, 2016). A single miRNA can regulate the expression of many genes and each mRNA can be targeted by multiple miRNAs, highlighting the complexity of miRNA biology.

## 1.4 microRNAs and Cancer

Calin et al. were the first to show involvement of aberrant miRNA expression in cancer progression (Calin et al., 2002). In fact, approximately half of all miRNAs were found to be located in "fragile sites," regions associated with cancer (Cummins & Velculescu, 2006) with ~73% of breast cancers exhibiting miRNA abnormalities (Zhang et al., 2006). Many studies have now shown miRNAs to function as both tumor suppressors and oncogenes (Bartel & Chen, 2004; Esquela-Kerscher & Slack, 2006; Nelson & Weiss, 2008) and have demonstrated that their dysregulation has implications in invasion, migration, and metastasis in breast cancer (Findlay, Turner, Moussa, & Watson, 2008; Huang et al., 2008; Iorio et al., 2005; Tavazoie et al., 2008). An example of an oncogenic miRNA is miR-21, that has been shown to be dysregulated in many cancers (Chan, Krichevsky, & Kosik, 2005; Slaby et al., 2007; Volinia et al., 2006; Yanaihara et al., 2006) including breast cancer (Iorio et al., 2005; Sempere et al., 2007). Clinically it has been reported that upregulation of miR-21 in primary breast cancer samples is associated with advanced clinical stage, lymph node metastasis, and poor prognosis (Yan et al., 2008). miR-21 has been shown to inhibit many tumor suppressor genes including TPM1 (Zhu, Si, Wu, & Mo, 2007), p53, PDCD4, and maspin (Zhu et al., 2008). An example of a tumor suppressive miRNA is miR-205, which was shown to be significantly downregulated in human breast tumors compared to matched normal (Wu, Zhu, & Mo, 2009). miR-205 suppresses cell proliferation, growth, and invasion by directly targeting HER3 and VEGF-A (Wang et al., 2013; Wu et al., 2009). It has also been shown to negatively regulate epithelial–mesenchymal transition (EMT) by targeting ZEB1 and ZEB2 (Gregory et al., 2008). Most recently, a group demonstrated that secretion of miR-205 from the tumor stroma promotes a cancer-associated stem cell phenotype which illustrates the importance of cellular and tissue context when studying miRNAs (Chao et al., 2014).

## 1.5 Circulating microRNAs

Recently, it was discovered that extracellular miRNAs circulate in the blood of both healthy and diseased patients, and they are both stable and detectable in human serum and plasma (Kosaka, Iguchi, & Ochiya, 2010; Kosaka, Iguchi, Yoshioka, et al., 2010). This allows miRNAs to be measured repeatedly and noninvasively and has sparked extensive research in miRNAs as therapeutic targets, as well as potential biomarkers of prognosis and diagnosis. The phenomenon of miRNA secretion and its role in intercellular communication has recently gained increased attention. Intensive studies have provided evidence that microvesicles, including exosomes, released from many cell types can transfer miRNAs to neighboring or distant cells, where these exogenous miRNAs function similarly to endogenous miRNAs to regulate target gene expression and recipient cell function (Kosaka, Iguchi, Yoshioka, et al., 2010; Mittelbrunn et al., 2011; Valadi et al., 2007). Therefore, secreted miRNAs may serve as a novel class of signaling molecules for mediating cell-to-cell communication.

### 1.6 microRNA Therapeutics

Currently, there are several companies involved in the development of therapeutically targeting microRNAs, either by overexpressing tumor suppressive miRNAs (Mirna Therapeutics) or by inhibiting oncomirs (Regulus Therapeutics). Mirna Therapeutics currently has a mimic of miR-34 in Phase I clinical trials for various solid tumors and hematological malignancies. Regulus Therapeutics has several anti-miRs in clinical trials for various diseases but the clinical initiative for oncology is still in the pre-clinical phase, but includes anti-miR to miR-21 which we described earlier is strongly associated with breast cancer.

## 2. microRNAs IN BREAST CANCER DISPARITIES

There continues to be controversy surrounding the impact of the biology of tumors from AA women driving aggressive breast cancer disease compared to the impact of socioeconomic factors that can result in higher mortality rates within this racial group. Several studies have shown that the increased mortality still exists in AA women with breast cancer after normalizing for these other factors (Albain et al., 2009; Bauer, Brown, Cress, Parise, & Caggiano, 2007; Lund et al., 2009). Therefore, studies have started to address what these biological differences might be and how they may influence not only the growth of these tumors, but how therapeutically they may be targeted differently. We know that all breast cancers are not the same and we are now beginning to understand the "same" subtype of breast cancer is not the same in women of different race. A pilot study in 2012 on African women in Nigeria with breast cancer showed that the biology was highly aggressive with high grade (III) and hormone receptor negative (65% TNBC) tumors as well as young age (mean age 47 years) at diagnosis (Adisa et al., 2012). This was a similar finding to that of others focused on women from Africa and other developing nations (Bird, Hill, & Houssami, 2008; Desai et al., 2000; Dey et al., 2009; Huo et al., 2009; Lokuhetty, Ranaweera, Wijeratne, Wickramasinghe, & Sheriffdeen, 2009; Mbonde, Amir, Akslen, & Kitinya, 2001; Yarney, Vanderpuye, & Clegg Lamptey, 2008). These studies argue toward more aggressive tumor biology in women of African descent independent of their location or other contributing factors.

There is little that is currently known about the role of microRNAs in breast cancer disparities. However, there are many ways in which a miRNA can be disparate in women with breast cancer (i) up- or downregulated miRNA in AA women; (ii) up- or downregulated gene that is known to be regulated/targeted by a disparate miRNA; (iii) presence of a SNP within a 3′UTR which abolishes or creates a miR-binding site; and (iv) the up- or downregulation of a disparate gene that contains an intronic miRNA. This review will highlight the miRNAs that are disparate that fall into these four categories, some of which overlap. We will also briefly mention published studies that are suggestive of potential disparities as areas of potential future development within the field.

A study in 2012 that performed gene expression profiling of benign tissue and malignant breast tumors from AA and CA women showed 23 differentially expressed genes between tumors and 13 between benign (Field et al., 2012). The genes that were found to be differentially regulated in the AA women are highlighted in Table 1 together with the miRNAs that have been experimentally validated to target them according to miRTarBase (Chou et al., 2016). Of interest the two genes in the signature (CRYBB2 and PSPHL) were also identified in this study as being disparate. However, in subsequent studies it was shown that AA women with invasive breast cancer are less likely (6%) to have deletion of the genome (7p11) where PSPHL resides (compared to 61% CA with invasive breast cancer). In addition, this study showed that the frequency of the deletion did not differ in AA women with and without invasive breast cancer, and that deletion of PSPHL was not associated with any pathological characteristics (Rummel, Penatzer, Shriver, & Ellsworth, 2014). Therefore, the authors concluded that elevated levels of PSPHL caused by retention of a 30 kb region of 7p11 in AA women does not contribute to cancer disparities, but instead represents population stratification. In contrast to this, another group independently identified both CRYBB2 and PSPHL as being disparate between AA and CA women with luminal A breast cancer

**Table 1** miRNAs That Are Validated to Target Differentially Regulated Genes in AA Women with Breast Cancer From the Ellsworth Group (Field et al., 2012)

| Gene Symbol | Gene Name | Up- or Downregulated in AA | Validated miRNAs | Intronic RNAs |
|---|---|---|---|---|
| SOS1 | Son of sevenless homolog 1 | Up | miR-124-3p | |
| COIL | Coilin | Up | miR-1-3p<br>let-7b-5p<br>miR-98-5p | |
| CRYBB2P1 | Crystalline beta B2 pseudogene 1 | Down | 0 | MIR6817 |
| EIF2S1 | Eukaryotic translation initiation | Down | miR-375 | |
| GOLPH3L | Golgi phosphoproteinn 3-like | Down | miR-16-5p<br>miR-15a-5p | |
| LTF | Lactotransferrin | Down | miR-214-3p | |
| RABEP1 | Rabaptin, RAB GTPase binding effector protein 1 | Down | miR-373-3p | |
| RYBP | RING1 and YY1 binding protein | Down | miR-9-5p | |
| ZNF395 | Zinc finger protein 395 | Down | miR-122-5p<br>miR-525-3p | |
| AR | Androgen receptor | Down | miR-488-5p,<br>miR-124-3p,<br>miR-185-5p,<br>miR-34a-5p,<br>miR-205-5p | |
| GPD1L | Glycerol-3-phosphate dehydrogenase 1-like | Down | miR-210-3p | |
| ABLIM1 | Actin-binding LIM protein 1 | Down | miR-34a-5p | |
| INSR | Insulin receptor | Down | miR-195-5p | |

Validated miRs are based on those annotated in miRTarBase 2016 with either one or more strong evidence and two or more less strong evidence (Chou et al., 2016).

(D'Arcy et al., 2015). These two genes were identified along with four others (ACOX2, MUC1, SQLE, and TYMS) that were differentially expressed and associated with survival (Table 2). For all six genes, tumors in AA had higher expression of poor prognosis genes (CRYBB2, PSPHL, SQLE, and TYMS) and lower expression of good prognosis genes (ACOX2 and MUC1). Similar to the previous study, this group also found PSPHL, along with CRYBB2, to be higher in AA normal tissue. However, their interpretation is that this may precede malignancy and contribute to mortality disparities.

As mentioned earlier, circulating microRNAs are of great interest due to their stability within bodily fluids, they have the potential as noninvasive biomarkers of early detection, diagnosis, treatment choice/response, and prognosis. Therefore, many studies have started exploring the differences in miRNA profiles in cancer, including the pilot study by Zhao et al., examining circulating miRNAs as potential biomarkers of early stage breast cancer (Zhao et al., 2010). Of interest, the study samples represented both AA and CA women with early stage breast cancer and race-matched controls. Microarray analysis showed that in women with early stage breast cancer, 9 miRNAs were up- and 9 were downregulated in AAs and 17 were up- and 14 were downregulated in CAs when compared to race-matched

**Table 2** miRNAs That Are Validated to Target Differentially Regulated Genes in AA Women with Luminal A Breast Cancer From the Troester Group (D'Arcy et al., 2015)

| Gene Symbol | Gene Name | Up- or Downregulated in AA | Validated miRNAs | Intronic RNAs |
|---|---|---|---|---|
| SQLE | Squalene epoxidase | Up | 0 | |
| TYMS | Thymidylate synthetase | Up | Let-7b-5p<br>miR-196a-5p<br>miR-433-3p | |
| ACOX2 | Acyl-CoA oxidase 2, branched chain | Down | miR-26b-5p | |
| MUC1 | Mucin 1, cell surface associated | Down | miR-145-5p<br>miR-1226-3p<br>miR-125b-5p<br>miR-124-3p<br>miR-455-3p | |

Validated miRs are based on those annotated in miRTarBase 2016 with either one or more strong evidence and two or more less strong evidence (Chou et al., 2016).

**Table 3** Circulating miRNAs That Are Uniquely Differentially Regulated in AA Women with Early Stage Breast Cancer (Zhao et al., 2010)

| microRNA Name | Genomic Location | Up- or Downregulated | Validated Target mRNAs | Intronic/ Intergenic |
|---|---|---|---|---|
| miR-425 | 3p21 | Up | CCND1 | DALRD3 |
| miR-483-5p | 11p15 | Up | SRF, MAPK3, FAM160B2, ALCAM | IGF2 |
| miR-485-3p | 14q32 | Up | NTRK3, NFYB, SLC40A1, MAT1A | Intergenic |
| miR-431 | 14q32 | Up | 0 | RTL1 (as) |
| miR-493 | 14q32 | Up | RHOC, MAP2K7, FZD4 | Intergenic |
| miR-558 | 2p22 | Up | 0 | BIRC6 |
| miR-331-5p | 12q22 | Up | 0 | Intergenic |
| miR-409-5p | 14q32 | Down | 0 | Intergenic |
| miR-642 | 19q13 | Down | DOHH | GIPR |
| miR-505 | Xq27 | Down | SRSF1 | ATP11C |
| miR-377 | 14q32 | Down | PPM1A, PAK1, SOD1, SOD2 | Intergenic |
| miR-340 | 5q35 | Down | MET | RNF130 |
| Let-7d | 9q22 | Down | HMGA2, APP, DICER, SLC11A2, PDGFA, IL13, MPL, EIF2C1, TNFRSF10B | Intergenic |

Genes that are validated targets of the identified miRNAs are based on those annotated in miRTarBase 2016 with either one or more strong evidence and two or more less strong evidence (Chou et al., 2016).

healthy controls, with only 2 miRNAs that overlapped between races (Table 3). These results, while preliminary, suggest that it might be necessary to develop race-specific circulating miRNA-based biomarkers in breast cancer early detection. It also suggests that there is validity to performing these same studies in different subtypes of breast cancer as well as in different stages of breast cancer.

Links between these dysregulated miRNAs and implications for breast cancer are highlighted later.

## 2.1 Upregulated in AA Women

*miR-425* was shown to be upregulated in AAs and has been shown to negatively regulate PTEN in breast cancer, a well-established tumor suppressor (Ahir et al., 2016). miR-425 was also shown to be expressed at high levels in breast cancer as part of a nine miRNA signature to detect ER+ breast cancer vs healthy controls (Kodahl et al., 2014). An interesting study in rats showed a downregulation of miR-425 in the mammary glands of once pregnant rats compared to virgin controls in the ALDH+ mammary epithelial cell population, which could suggest an anticarcinogenic or protective role after pregnancy (Nandy et al., 2014). Some studies also suggest its tumor suppressor function, but we highlight here the effects on tumor promotion.

*miR-483-5p* was shown to be upregulated in cisplatin resistant tongue squamous cell carcinoma (Fan et al., 2015). This could have implications for breast cancer as platinum agents are used to treat TNBC patients, especially as this subtype is more prevalent in AA women, and this study also showed that high levels of miR-483-5p led to poor/lower overall survival (OS) (Fan et al., 2015). Elevated levels of miR-483 were also observed in higher stages (III and IV vs I and II) of ovarian cancer (Zheng et al., 2013). This has implications for cancer disparities as ovarian cancer mortality rates are higher in AA women (American Cancer Society, 2016).

*miR-485-3p* is generally considered to be a tumor suppressor in breast cancer (Anaya-Ruiz, Bandala, & Perez-Santos, 2013; He et al., 2014; Lou et al., 2016), but is part of a cluster of miRNAs that are dysregulated in chromosomal region 14q32 that have been implicated in cancer.

*miR-431* has no published studies directly related to breast cancer, however, elevated levels have been shown to distinguish stage IV colorectal cancer from controls as part of a three circulating miRNA signature (Kanaan et al., 2013). Elevated levels have also been shown to be upregulated in vestibular schwannomas when compared to control nerves (Torres-Martin et al., 2013) and are correlated with OS in pancreatic cancer patients (Schultz et al., 2012). This same pancreatic study showed that miR-431 expression ranked sixth out of nine in the strongest predictive abilities for OS and 5th out of 14 in 2-year follow up. Decreased levels have been shown to inhibit cellular proliferation in glioblastoma by upregulation of its direct target SOCS6 and subsequent suppression of the JAK-STAT signaling pathway (Tanaka et al., 2014).

*miR-493* is upregulated in male breast cancer (Lehmann et al., 2010). High levels are also associated with resistance to microtubule drugs (e.g., paclitaxel), advanced forms of ovarian cancer, and reduced survival of ovarian and breast cancer patients with aggressive tumors (Tambe et al., 2016). This study also suggested that intratumoral profiling of miR-493 could have diagnostic value in predicting the efficacy to taxane chemotherapy. In TNBC, miR-493 is part of a four miRNA signature that allowed subdivision of TNBCs into high and low risk groups. They were also able to clearly identify worse outcome patients in the treated and untreated subcohorts, therefore having both diagnostic and prognostic value (Gasparini et al., 2014).

*miR-558* has no published studies directly related to breast cancer, however it has been shown to be upregulated in neuroblastoma (Qu et al., 2015; Shohet et al., 2011) and upregulated in response to high doses of radiation in fibroblasts (Maes, An, Sarojini, Wu, & Wang, 2008). This could have implications in the tumor microenvironment as outlined in Section 3.

*miR-331-5p* has no published studies directly related to breast cancer, however elevated levels in colorectal cancer patients, as part of an eight miRNA signature, can distinguish polyps from controls with high accuracy (Verma et al., 2015). Elevated circulating levels are correlated with hepatocarcinogenic progression in rats (Sukata et al., 2011). Elevated levels are found in acute and chronic lymphocytic leukemia (Zanette et al., 2007) but in acute myeloid leukemia downregulated miR-331-5p is associated with worse response to therapy and shorter survival (Butrym et al., 2015).

## 2.2 Downregulated in AA Women

*miR-409-5p* has no published studies directly related to breast cancer, however stromal-derived miR-409 was shown to drive EMT and tumorigenesis in prostate cancer (Josson et al., 2015). The most well-studied form of this miRNA is the 3p arm (miR-409-3p). miR-409 is located on chromosome 14q32 along with miR-377 which is also downregulated in AA women. Allelic deletions of this region are frequently observed in breast cancer (Kerangueven et al., 1997).

*miR-642* has no published studies directly related to breast cancer, however upregulated levels are associated with increased sensitivity to cisplatin in bladder cancer cell lines (Nordentoft et al., 2012), which has potential implications for cisplatin resistance in AA breast cancer patients. miR-642 is downregulated in prostate cancer cell lines compared to normal prostate and upregulation decreased proliferation and the levels of its host gene (DOHH). In prostate cancer patients, the levels of miR-642 and DOHH were inversely correlated (Epis et al., 2012).

*miR-505* was identified as part of a six miRNA signature to discriminate BRCA mutation carriers from noncarriers with 92% accuracy (Tanic et al., 2015). This could have implications for disparities based on the lower occurrence of BRCA1 mutation carriers in AA women. Circulating levels of miR-505 were shown to be upregulated in pretreated breast cancer patients compared to healthy controls (Matamala et al., 2015). This is contrary to the reported decreased levels of miR-505 in breast tumor tissue suggesting miR-505 as a tumor suppressive miRNA (Yamamoto et al., 2011). However, this is not unusual as intratumoral levels and circulating levels within the same patient have been shown to not always positively correlate. This study reported the genomic deletion of miR-505 in adriamycin-resistant MCF7 cells (MCF7/ADR), suggesting its role in conferring sensitivity to adriamycin. This could have implications for treatment choice for AA women with breast cancer. Interestingly, the study showing elevated circulating miR-505 levels in pretreated patients also reported its decrease in a group of treated patients (Matamala et al., 2015). Elevated miR-505 levels have been shown to strongly and significantly correlate to high proliferation, ER negativity, and cytokeratin 5/6 positivity in lymph node negative breast cancers (Jonsdottir et al., 2012). These data together support the potential utility of miR-505 to monitor treatment response and highlight its potential clinical value as a noninvasive biomarker for breast cancer detection, typing, and surveillance.

*miR-377* was identified as part of a four miRNA signature to identify PR+ status in breast cancer (Lowery et al., 2009). A positive correlation was also observed between miR-377 and recurrence score (RS) from Oncotype DX® (Emmadi et al., 2015). Oncotype DX® testing is for treatment stratification of ER+, lymph node negative breast cancers. The RS is represented by a number 0–100, which correlates to a specific likelihood of breast cancer recurrence within 10 years of initial diagnosis (Paik et al., 2006).

*miR-340* has been shown to inhibit migration, invasion, and metastasis of breast cancer by targeting the wnt pathway (Mohammadi-Yeganeh et al., 2016), MYO10 (Chen et al., 2016), and c-met (Wu et al., 2011). Similar to that described earlier for miR-505, miR-340 can distinguish BRCA1 mutation carriers from noncarriers (Tanic et al., 2015). miR-340 loss has been associated with lymph node metastasis, high tumor histological grade, clinical stage, and shorter OS in breast cancer tissue specimens (Wu et al., 2011).

*Let-7d* expression is correlated with better OS in the ER−/HER2− subtype of breast cancer (Lee et al., 2016). In the hallmark study, characterizing the miRNAs that are dysregulated during breast cancer progression, let-7d was shown to be downregulated during the transition from normal to DCIS and then upregulated during the transition from in situ to invasive breast cancer (Volinia et al., 2012). It has also been shown that LIN28 promotes tumorigenic activity by suppressing let-7d miRNA maturation in breast cancer cells (Sakurai et al., 2012).

The Singh group recently performed cytokine profiling in serum samples from AA and CA breast cancer patients and identified resistin (RETN) and IL-6 as being elevated in AA women (Deshmukh et al., 2015). Although there are no known miRNAs that are validated to target resistin, several have been validated for IL-6 (miR-223-3p, let7a-5p, miR-203a-3p, miR-142-3p, miR-26a-5p, miR-365a-3p, miR-107, let-7c-5p, and miR-149-5p) and although none of these have been specifically linked to be disparate in breast cancer there are many other miRNAs that are predicted to target both of these genes that may be disparate including miR-505, which as described earlier is downregulated in the circulation of AA women with breast cancer and is predicted to target RETN (Agarwal, Bell, Nam, & Bartel, 2015).

Tamoxifen sensitivity varies among breast cancer patients and ~35% of patients are reported to not respond (Clarke, Leonessa, Welch, & Skaar, 2001). In addition, although AA women are less likely to get ER+ breast cancer compared to CA women, most of the pharmacogenomics research on tamoxifen therapy has been conducted in patients of Caucasian ancestry. Therefore, a study was performed to evaluate genetic variants related to tamoxifen therapy in African-derived samples (Weng, Ziliak, Lacroix, Geeleher, & Huang, 2014). This study used an integrative "omic" analysis for tamoxifen sensitivity and identified 50 single nucleotide polymorphisms (SNPs) that were associated with cellular sensitivity to endoxifen (an active metabolite of tamoxifen) through their effects on 34 genes and 30 miRNAs. Of the SNPs identified some were common to both ancestries but others were unique to the African samples, warranting further study.

Another group examined genetic variants in 145 SNPs in 6 miRNA processing genes and 78 miRNAs whose targets are important for breast cancer between AA and CA women and observed that the allele frequencies of most (87%) of the SNPs differed significantly by race (Yao et al., 2013). Of note, no associations were observed in both the AA and CA populations. However, one limitation of the study was a lack of a validation population and therefore further study is needed to validate the findings and to explore the genetic basis and underlying mechanisms of the associations. The Carolina Breast Cancer study also investigated association of germline microRNA SNPs in pre-miRNA flanking regions and breast cancer risk and survival among AA and CA women (Bensen et al., 2013). They genotyped nine SNPs within six pre-miRNA gene sequences and found two miR-185 SNPs, rs2008591 and rs887205, that were inversely associated with breast cancer risk in AA women. They also identified two SNPs, rs4938723 in miR-34b/34c and rrs6920648 in miR-20b that were associated with breast cancer survival overall. Similar to the previous SNP study described further validation is required to confirm these findings.

## 3. microRNAs IN TUMOR MICROENVIRONMENT

The impact and significance of the tumor microenvironment (or stroma) on tumor biology is becoming increasingly clear. Many studies are now focused on the different cellular types within the stroma, including immune cells, fibroblasts, and endothelial cells and their impact on tumor "epithelial" cells. However again, few studies have assessed the tumor microenvironment and how it might differ between women of different race. The Nigerian study mentioned earlier also reported a high infiltration of tumor-associated macrophages (TAMs) in these tumors (Adisa et al., 2012). The occurrence of high numbers of macrophages in the tumor stroma has been associated with tumor progression and poor prognosis in breast and other solid malignancies. Tissue sections were stained with CD68 plus PCNA, which marks a subset of TAMs that have been shown to be associated with poor outcomes in breast cancer (Campbell et al., 2011; Mukhtar et al., 2011). They found that 82% of the cases had high levels of CD68/PCNA positive TAMs and that they were more prevalent in hormone receptor (HR) negative or triple-negative cases, compared to hormone receptor positive cases. A second marker, Mac387, was also used and they found 65% of the cases had high numbers of Mac387 cells. As with the CD68/PCNA TAMs, Mac387 cells were most prevalent in HR- or triple-negative tumors. Since then, a study was published showing that macrophage numbers were significantly higher in tumors from AA (90% positive) and Latina (89% positive) than in Caucasian women (40% positive) in the United States (Carrio et al., 2013), although in this study they only used a single marker to identify the TAMs (CD68) and this study was performed in small ER+ breast cancers.

A study looking at the normal breast microenvironment of premenopausal women found that the fibroblasts from AA and CA women differentially influenced the behavior of breast cancer cells both in vitro and in vivo (Fleming et al., 2010). Whole breast extracellular matrix (ECM) was isolated from CA and AA women and they found that ER−/PR− cells were significantly more aggressive when in contact with AA ECM. In contrast ER+/PR+ cells were more aggressive with CA ECM contact. They also performed mass spectrometry of the isolated ECM and showed that only 22% of the proteins that were identified were in common. Of interest, the AA proteins associated with breast cancer that they identified were primarily related to tumorigenesis/neoplasia, while CA unique proteins were involved with growth/metastasis.

A study was published in 2009 looking at the tumor microenvironment differences between AA and CA women with breast cancer (Martin et al., 2009). They performed genome-wide mRNA expression analysis specific to the tumor epithelium and stroma and found that many genes were differentially regulated between them. Very few miRNAs that target these genes have been validated (highlighted in Table 4) but it could be of particular interest therapeutically to identify the miRNAs that target these disparately regulated genes.

Of interest, gene ontology and disease association analyses indicated that pathways related to tumor angiogenesis and chemotaxis could be functionally different between AA and CA women and they further demonstrated higher levels of microvessel density and TAMs in AA tumors, which closely matches the studies described earlier. The authors had previously shown that PSPHL and CRYBB2 could be used as a two gene classifier to differentiate between AA and CA prostate cancer patients (Wallace et al., 2008). Therefore, to test if similar signatures exist in breast cancer, they applied the same prediction analysis and found that the two gene signature could also distinguish between the breast tumor epithelia from AA (94%) and CA (100%) women. They confirmed this result in 55 additional breast tumors (27 AA and 28 CA) and correctly classified 93% of the AA patients and 86% of the CA patients.

The inhibition of let-7d in epithelial cells, one of the miRNAs that was shown to be downregulated in the circulation of AA women with breast cancer, has been shown to cause changes associated with an EMT when inhibited both in vitro and in vivo (Willis et al., 2005). A study then focused on whether the expression of let-7d in fibroblasts was able to alter their mesenchymal features. They showed that expression of let-7d was able to decrease mesenchymal markers α-smooth muscle actin, N-cadherin, fibroblast-specific protein-1 and fibronectin, as well as increase in epithelial

**Table 4** miRNAs That Are Validated to Target Differentially Regulated Genes in AA Women with Breast Cancer From the Ambs Group (Martin et al., 2009)

| Gene Symbol | Gene Name | Up- or Downregulated in AA | Validated miRNAs | Intronic miRNAs |
|---|---|---|---|---|
| PSPHP1 (PSPHL) | Phosphoserine phosphatase pseudogene 1 | Up (Epithelium and Stroma) | 0 | |
| AMFR | Autocrine motility factor receptor | Up (Epithelium) | miR-376a-5p, miR-29a/b/c-3p | |
| EDG2 (LPAR1) | Lysophosphatidic acid receptor 1 | Down (Epithelium) | miR-200c-3p, miR-23a-3p | |
| CXCL10 | C-X-C motif chemokine ligand 10 | Up (Stroma) | miR-21 | |
| SLC38A1 | Solute carrier family 38 member 1 | Up (Stroma) | miR-16-5p, miR-30a-5p | |
| PSMA2 | Proteasome subunit alpha 2 | Up (Stroma) | miR-132-3p | |
| LASS6 (CERS6) | Ceramide synthase 6 | Up (Stroma) | 0 | MIR4774 |
| SOS1 | SOS Ras/Rac guanine nucleotide exchange factor 1 | Up (Stroma) | miR-124-3p | |
| ARF4 | ATP ribosylation factor 4 | Up (Stroma) | miR-1-3p, miR-7-5p | |
| GGCT (C7orf24) | Gamma-glutamylcyclotransferase | Up (Stroma) | Let-7b-5p | |
| PTRF | Polymerase 1 and transcript release factor | Down (Stroma) | miR-124-3p | |
| NUAK1 | NUAK family kinase 1 | Down (Stroma) | miR-211-5p | |
| AQP1 | Aquaporin 1 | Down (Stroma) | miR-320a | |

Validated miRs are based on those annotated in miRTarBase 2016 with either one or more strong evidence and two or more less strong evidence (Chou et al., 2016).

markers tight junction protein-1 and keratin 19 (Huleihel et al., 2014). They further went on to show that let-7d expression could phenotypically alter fibroblasts including delaying wound healing and reducing mobility and proliferation. This has implications for the activation of fibroblasts in the tumor microenvironment to cancer-associated fibroblasts which are known to promote aggressive tumor growth and metastasis (Qiao, Gu, Guo, Zhang, & Fu, 2016). Let-7d has also been shown to suppress growth, metastasis, and tumor macrophage infiltration in renal cell carcinoma (Su et al., 2014), suggesting that the loss of let-7d in AA women has implications for the entire tumor population of cells not just the epithelium.

## 4. SUMMARY AND FUTURE PERSPECTIVES

Although a few studies have begun to investigate the potential role of miRNAs in breast cancer disparities, there is still a lot that is currently unknown. However, it is clear from a review of the literature that we are beginning to understand that miRNAs are a major player in the dysregulation that occurs in women leading to the initiation and progression of breast cancer. It is also clear that the tumor biology of breast cancer in women can differ not only by subtype but by race, explaining, at least in part, the increased mortality observed in AA women with breast cancer. Although there are many issues that can lead to an increase in mortality, and it is critical that these are addressed, one can no longer argue that the tumor biology between different racial groups is the same. If we hope to reduce breast cancer disparities, we must make a concerted effort to study the differences in tumor biology so that we may reduce mortality rates in all women. This information is critical if we want to address the problem of breast cancer and develop treatment strategies with a personalized medicine approach.

## ACKNOWLEDGMENT

This work was supported in part by the NIH SC CaDRe P20 CA157066-01A1 grant.

## REFERENCES

Adisa, C. A., Eleweke, N., Alfred, A. A., Campbell, M. J., Sharma, R., Nseyo, O., … Esserman, L. J. (2012). Biology of breast cancer in Nigerian women: A pilot study. *Annals of African Medicine*, *11*(3), 169–175. http://dx.doi.org/10.4103/1596-3519.96880. AnnAfrMed_2012_11_3_169_96880 [pii].

Agarwal, V., Bell, G. W., Nam, J. W., & Bartel, D. P. (2015). Predicting effective microRNA target sites in mammalian mRNAs. *eLife*, *4*, 1–38. http://dx.doi.org/10.7554/eLife.05005.

Ahir, M., Bhattacharya, S., Karmakar, S., Mukhopadhyay, A., Mukherjee, S., Ghosh, S., … Adhikary, A. (2016). Tailored-CuO-nanowire decorated with folic acid mediated coupling of the mitochondrial-ROS generation and miR425-PTEN axis in furnishing potent anti-cancer activity in human triple negative breast carcinoma cells. *Biomaterials*, *76*, 115–132. http://dx.doi.org/10.1016/j.biomaterials.2015.10.044. S0142-9612(15)00854-6 [pii].

Albain, K. S., Unger, J. M., Crowley, J. J., Coltman, C. A., Jr., & Hershman, D. L. (2009). Racial disparities in cancer survival among randomized clinical trials patients of the Southwest Oncology Group. *Journal of the National Cancer Institute*, *101*(14), 984–992. http://dx.doi.org/10.1093/jnci/djp175. djp175 [pii].

Ali, S., Mondal, N., Choudhry, H., Rasool, M., Pushparaj, P. N., Khan, M. A., … Jamal, M. S. (2016). Current management strategies in breast cancer by targeting key altered molecular players. *Frontiers in Oncology*, *6*, 45. http://dx.doi.org/10.3389/fonc.2016.00045.

Ambros, V. (2004). The functions of animal microRNAs. *Nature*, *431*(7006), 350–355. http://dx.doi.org/10.1038/nature02871. nature02871 [pii].

American Cancer Society. (2016). *Cancer facts & figures 2016*. Atlanta, GA: American Cancer Society.

Anaya-Ruiz, M., Bandala, C., & Perez-Santos, J. L. (2013). miR-485 acts as a tumor suppressor by inhibiting cell growth and migration in breast carcinoma T47D cells. *Asian Pacific Journal of Cancer Prevention*, *14*(6), 3757–3760.

Bartel, D. P. (2004). MicroRNAs: Genomics, biogenesis, mechanism, and function. *Cell*, *116*(2), 281–297. http://dx.doi.org/S0092867404000455. [pii].

Bartel, D. P., & Chen, C. Z. (2004). Micromanagers of gene expression: The potentially widespread influence of metazoan microRNAs. *Nature Reviews. Genetics*, *5*(5), 396–400. http://dx.doi.org/10.1038/nrg1328. nrg1328 [pii].

Bauer, K. R., Brown, M., Cress, R. D., Parise, C. A., & Caggiano, V. (2007). Descriptive analysis of estrogen receptor (ER)-negative, progesterone receptor (PR)-negative, and HER2-negative invasive breast cancer, the so-called triple-negative phenotype: A population-based study from the California cancer Registry. *Cancer*, *109*(9), 1721–1728. http://dx.doi.org/10.1002/cncr.22618.

Bensen, J. T., Tse, C. K., Nyante, S. J., Barnholtz-Sloan, J. S., Cole, S. R., & Millikan, R. C. (2013). Association of germline microRNA SNPs in pre-miRNA flanking region and breast cancer risk and survival: The Carolina Breast Cancer Study. *Cancer Causes & Control*, *24*(6), 1099–1109. http://dx.doi.org/10.1007/s10552-013-0187-z.

Bird, P. A., Hill, A. G., & Houssami, N. (2008). Poor hormone receptor expression in East African breast cancer: Evidence of a biologically different disease? *Annals of Surgical Oncology*, *15*(7), 1983–1988. http://dx.doi.org/10.1245/s10434-008-9900-7.

Butrym, A., Rybka, J., Baczynska, D., Tukiendorf, A., Kuliczkowski, K., & Mazur, G. (2015). Expression of microRNA-331 can be used as a predictor for response to therapy and survival in acute myeloid leukemia patients. *Biomarkers in Medicine*, *9*(5), 453–460. http://dx.doi.org/10.2217/bmm.14.112.

Calin, G. A., Dumitru, C. D., Shimizu, M., Bichi, R., Zupo, S., Noch, E., … Croce, C. M. (2002). Frequent deletions and down-regulation of micro- RNA genes miR15 and miR16 at 13q14 in chronic lymphocytic leukemia. *Proceedings of the National Academy of Sciences of the United States of America*, *99*(24), 15524–15529. http://dx.doi.org/10.1073/pnas.242606799. 242606799 [pii].

Campbell, M. J., Tonlaar, N. Y., Garwood, E. R., Huo, D., Moore, D. H., Khramtsov, A. I., … Esserman, L. J. (2011). Proliferating macrophages associated with high grade, hormone receptor negative breast cancer and poor clinical outcome. *Breast Cancer Research and Treatment*, *128*(3), 703–711. http://dx.doi.org/10.1007/s10549-010-1154-y.

Carrio, R., Koru-Sengul, T., Miao, F., Gluck, S., Lopez, O., Selman, Y., ... Torroella-Kouri, M. (2013). Macrophages as independent prognostic factors in small T1 breast cancers. *Oncology Reports*, *29*(1), 141–148. http://dx.doi.org/10.3892/or.2012.2088.

Chan, J. A., Krichevsky, A. M., & Kosik, K. S. (2005). MicroRNA-21 is an antiapoptotic factor in human glioblastoma cells. *Cancer Research*, *65*(14), 6029–6033. http://dx.doi.org/10.1158/0008-5472.CAN-05-0137. 65/14/6029 [pii].

Chao, C. H., Chang, C. C., Wu, M. J., Ko, H. W., Wang, D., Hung, M. C., ... Chang, C. J. (2014). MicroRNA-205 signaling regulates mammary stem cell fate and tumorigenesis. *The Journal of Clinical Investigation*, *124*(7), 3093–3106. http://dx.doi.org/10.1172/JCI73351. 73351 [pii].

Chen, C. P., Sun, Z. L., Lu, X., Wu, W. X., Guo, W. L., Lu, J. J., ... Fang, Y. (2016). miR-340 suppresses cell migration and invasion by targeting MYO10 in breast cancer. *Oncology Reports*, *35*(2), 709–716. http://dx.doi.org/10.3892/or.2015.4411.

Chou, C. H., Chang, N. W., Shrestha, S., Hsu, S. D., Lin, Y. L., Lee, W. H., ... Huang, H. D. (2016). miRTarBase 2016: Updates to the experimentally validated miRNA–target interactions database. *Nucleic Acids Research*, *44*(D1), D239–D247. http://dx.doi.org/10.1093/nar/gkv1258. gkv1258 [pii].

Clarke, R., Leonessa, F., Welch, J. N., & Skaar, T. C. (2001). Cellular and molecular pharmacology of antiestrogen action and resistance. *Pharmacological Reviews*, *53*(1), 25–71.

Cummins, J. M., & Velculescu, V. E. (2006). Implications of micro-RNA profiling for cancer diagnosis. *Oncogene*, *25*(46), 6220–6227. http://dx.doi.org/10.1038/sj.onc.1209914. 1209914 [pii].

D'Arcy, M., Fleming, J., Robinson, W. R., Kirk, E. L., Perou, C. M., & Troester, M. A. (2015). Race-associated biological differences among Luminal A breast tumors. *Breast Cancer Research and Treatment*, *152*(2), 437–448. http://dx.doi.org/10.1007/s10549-015-3474-4.

Desai, S. B., Moonim, M. T., Gill, A. K., Punia, R. S., Naresh, K. N., & Chinoy, R. F. (2000). Hormone receptor status of breast cancer in India: A study of 798 tumours. *Breast*, *9*(5), 267–270. http://dx.doi.org/10.1054/brst.2000.0134. discussion 270. S0960-9776(00)90134-6 [pii].

DeSantis, C. E., Siegel, R. L., Sauer, A. G., Miller, K. D., Fedewa, S. A., Alcaraz, K. I., & Jemal, A. (2016). Cancer statistics for African Americans, 2016: Progress and opportunities in reducing racial disparities. *CA: A Cancer Journal for Clinicians*, *66*(4), 290–308. http://dx.doi.org/10.3322/caac.21340.

Deshmukh, S. K., Srivastava, S. K., Bhardwaj, A., Singh, A. P., Tyagi, N., Marimuthu, S., ... Singh, S. (2015). Resistin and interleukin-6 exhibit racially-disparate expression in breast cancer patients, display molecular association and promote growth and aggressiveness of tumor cells through STAT3 activation. *Oncotarget*, *6*(13), 11231–11241. http://dx.doi.org/10.18632/oncotarget.3591. 3591 [pii].

Dey, S., Boffetta, P., Mathews, A., Brennan, P., Soliman, A., & Mathew, A. (2009). Risk factors according to estrogen receptor status of breast cancer patients in Trivandrum, South India. *International Journal of Cancer*, *125*(7), 1663–1670. http://dx.doi.org/10.1002/ijc.24460.

Emmadi, R., Canestrari, E., Arbieva, Z. H., Mu, W., Dai, Y., Frasor, J., & Wiley, E. (2015). Correlative analysis of miRNA expression and oncotype Dx recurrence score in estrogen receptor positive breast carcinomas. *PLoS One*, *10*(12), e0145346. http://dx.doi.org/10.1371/journal.pone.0145346. PONE-D-15-37080 [pii].

Epis, M. R., Giles, K. M., Kalinowski, F. C., Barker, A., Cohen, R. J., & Leedman, P. J. (2012). Regulation of expression of deoxyhypusine hydroxylase (DOHH), the enzyme that catalyzes the activation of eIF5A, by miR-331-3p and miR-642-5p in prostate cancer cells. *The Journal of Biological Chemistry*, *287*(42), 35251–35259. http://dx.doi.org/10.1074/jbc.M112.374686. M112.374686 [pii].

Esquela-Kerscher, A., & Slack, F. J. (2006). Oncomirs—microRNAs with a role in cancer. *Nature Reviews. Cancer*, *6*(4), 259–269. http://dx.doi.org/10.1038/nrc1840. nrc1840 [pii].

Fan, S., Chen, W. X., Lv, X. B., Tang, Q. L., Sun, L. J., Liu, B. D., … Li, J. S. (2015). miR-483-5p determines mitochondrial fission and cisplatin sensitivity in tongue squamous cell carcinoma by targeting FIS1. *Cancer Letters*, *362*(2), 183–191. http://dx.doi.org/10.1016/j.canlet.2015.03.045. S0304-3835(15)00247-5 [pii].

Field, L. A., Love, B., Deyarmin, B., Hooke, J. A., Shriver, C. D., & Ellsworth, R. E. (2012). Identification of differentially expressed genes in breast tumors from African American compared with Caucasian women. *Cancer*, *118*(5), 1334–1344. http://dx.doi.org/10.1002/cncr.26405.

Findlay, V. J., Turner, D. P., Moussa, O., & Watson, D. K. (2008). MicroRNA-mediated inhibition of prostate-derived Ets factor messenger RNA translation affects prostate-derived Ets factor regulatory networks in human breast cancer. *Cancer Research*, *68*(20), 8499–8506. http://dx.doi.org/10.1158/0008-5472.CAN-08-0907. 68/20/8499 [pii].

Fleming, J. M., Miller, T. C., Quinones, M., Xiao, Z., Xu, X., Meyer, M. J., … Vonderhaar, B. K. (2010). The normal breast microenvironment of premenopausal women differentially influences the behavior of breast cancer cells in vitro and in vivo. *BMC Medicine*, *8*, 27. http://dx.doi.org/10.1186/1741-7015-8-27. 1741-7015-8-27 [pii].

Gasparini, P., Cascione, L., Fassan, M., Lovat, F., Guler, G., Balci, S., … Huebner, K. (2014). microRNA expression profiling identifies a four microRNA signature as a novel diagnostic and prognostic biomarker in triple negative breast cancers. *Oncotarget*, *5*(5), 1174–1184. http://dx.doi.org/10.18632/oncotarget.1682. 1682 [pii].

Gregory, P. A., Bert, A. G., Paterson, E. L., Barry, S. C., Tsykin, A., Farshid, G., … Goodall, G. J. (2008). The miR-200 family and miR-205 regulate epithelial to mesenchymal transition by targeting ZEB1 and SIP1. *Nature Cell Biology*, *10*(5), 593–601. http://dx.doi.org/10.1038/ncb1722. ncb1722 [pii].

He, L., & Hannon, G. J. (2004). MicroRNAs: Small RNAs with a big role in gene regulation. *Nature Reviews. Genetics*, *5*(7), 522–531. http://dx.doi.org/10.1038/nrg1379. nrg1379 [pii].

He, N., Zheng, H., Li, P., Zhao, Y., Zhang, W., Song, F., & Chen, K. (2014). miR-485-5p binding site SNP rs8752 in HPGD gene is associated with breast cancer risk. *PLoS One*, *9*(7), e102093. http://dx.doi.org/10.1371/journal.pone.0102093. PONE-D-14-04389 [pii].

Huang, Q., Gumireddy, K., Schrier, M., le Sage, C., Nagel, R., Nair, S., … Agami, R. (2008). The microRNAs miR-373 and miR-520c promote tumour invasion and metastasis. *Nature Cell Biology*, *10*(2), 202–210. http://dx.doi.org/10.1038/ncb1681. ncb1681 [pii].

Huleihel, L., Ben-Yehudah, A., Milosevic, J., Yu, G., Pandit, K., Sakamoto, K., … Kaminski, N. (2014). Let-7d microRNA affects mesenchymal phenotypic properties of lung fibroblasts. *American Journal of Physiology. Lung Cellular and Molecular Physiology*, *306*(6), L534–L542. http://dx.doi.org/10.1152/ajplung.00149.2013. ajplung.00149.2013 [pii].

Huo, D., Ikpatt, F., Khramtsov, A., Dangou, J. M., Nanda, R., Dignam, J., … Olopade, O. I. (2009). Population differences in breast cancer: Survey in indigenous African women reveals over-representation of triple-negative breast cancer. *Journal of Clinical Oncology*, *27*(27), 4515–4521. http://dx.doi.org/10.1200/JCO.2008.19.6873. JCO.2008.19.6873 [pii].

Inoue, K., & Fry, E. A. (2016). Novel molecular markers for breast cancer. *Biomarkers in Cancer*, *8*, 25–42. http://dx.doi.org/10.4137/BIC.S38394.

Iorio, M. V., Ferracin, M., Liu, C. G., Veronese, A., Spizzo, R., Sabbioni, S., … Croce, C. M. (2005). MicroRNA gene expression deregulation in human breast cancer. *Cancer Research*, *65*(16), 7065–7070. http://dx.doi.org/10.1158/0008-5472.CAN-05-1783. doi: 65/16/7065 [pii].

Jonsdottir, K., Janssen, S. R., Da Rosa, F. C., Gudlaugsson, E., Skaland, I., Baak, J. P., & Janssen, E. A. (2012). Validation of expression patterns for nine miRNAs in 204 lymph-node negative breast cancers. *PLoS One*, 7(11), e48692. http://dx.doi.org/10.1371/journal.pone.0048692. PONE-D-12-19715 [pii].

Josson, S., Gururajan, M., Sung, S. Y., Hu, P., Shao, C., Zhau, H. E., … Chung, L. W. (2015). Stromal fibroblast-derived miR-409 promotes epithelial-to-mesenchymal transition and prostate tumorigenesis. *Oncogene*, *34*(21), 2690–2699. http://dx.doi.org/10.1038/onc.2014.212. onc2014212 [pii].

Kanaan, Z., Roberts, H., Eichenberger, M. R., Billeter, A., Ocheretner, G., Pan, J., … Galandiuk, S. (2013). A plasma microRNA panel for detection of colorectal adenomas: A step toward more precise screening for colorectal cancer. *Annals of Surgery*, *258*(3), 400–408. http://dx.doi.org/10.1097/SLA.0b013e3182a15bcc. 00000658-201309000-00004 [pii].

Kent, O. A., & Mendell, J. T. (2006). A small piece in the cancer puzzle: microRNAs as tumor suppressors and oncogenes. *Oncogene*, *25*(46), 6188–6196. http://dx.doi.org/10.1038/sj.onc.1209913. 1209913 [pii].

Kerangueven, F., Noguchi, T., Coulier, F., Allione, F., Wargniez, V., Simony-Lafontaine, J., … Birnbaum, D. (1997). Genome-wide search for loss of heterozygosity shows extensive genetic diversity of human breast carcinomas. *Cancer Research*, *57*(24), 5469–5474.

Kittaneh, M., Montero, A. J., & Gluck, S. (2013). Molecular profiling for breast cancer: A comprehensive review. *Biomarkers in Cancer*, *5*, 61–70. http://dx.doi.org/10.4137/BIC.S9455. bic-5-2013-061 [pii].

Kodahl, A. R., Lyng, M. B., Binder, H., Cold, S., Gravgaard, K., Knoop, A. S., & Ditzel, H. J. (2014). Novel circulating microRNA signature as a potential non-invasive multi-marker test in ER-positive early-stage breast cancer: A case control study. *Molecular Oncology*, *8*(5), 874–883. http://dx.doi.org/10.1016/j.molonc.2014.03.002. S1574-7891(14)00050-7 [pii].

Kosaka, N., Iguchi, H., & Ochiya, T. (2010a). Circulating microRNA in body fluid: A new potential biomarker for cancer diagnosis and prognosis. *Cancer Science*, *101*(10), 2087–2092. http://dx.doi.org/10.1111/j.1349-7006.2010.01650.x. CAS1650 [pii].

Kosaka, N., Iguchi, H., Yoshioka, Y., Takeshita, F., Matsuki, Y., & Ochiya, T. (2010b). Secretory mechanisms and intercellular transfer of microRNAs in living cells. *The Journal of Biological Chemistry*, *285*(23), 17442–17452. http://dx.doi.org/10.1074/jbc.M110.107821. M110.107821 [pii].

Lee, E., Ito, K., Zhao, Y., Schadt, E. E., Irie, H. Y., & Zhu, J. (2016). Inferred miRNA activity identifies miRNA-mediated regulatory networks underlying multiple cancers. *Bioinformatics*, *32*(1), 96–105. http://dx.doi.org/10.1093/bioinformatics/btv531. btv531 [pii].

Lehmann, U., Streichert, T., Otto, B., Albat, C., Hasemeier, B., Christgen, H., … Langer, F. (2010). Identification of differentially expressed microRNAs in human male breast cancer. *BMC Cancer*, *10*, 109. http://dx.doi.org/10.1186/1471-2407-10-109. 1471-2407-10-109 [pii].

Lokuhetty, M. D., Ranaweera, G. G., Wijeratne, M. D., Wickramasinghe, K. H., & Sheriffdeen, A. H. (2009). Profile of breast cancer in a group of women in a developing country in South Asia: Is there a difference? *World Journal of Surgery*, *33*(3), 455–459. http://dx.doi.org/10.1007/s00268-008-9860-x.

Lou, C., Xiao, M., Cheng, S., Lu, X., Jia, S., Ren, Y., & Li, Z. (2016). MiR-485-3p and miR-485-5p suppress breast cancer cell metastasis by inhibiting PGC-1alpha expression. *Cell Death & Disease*, 7, e2159. http://dx.doi.org/10.1038/cddis.2016.27. cddis201627 [pii].

Lowery, A. J., Miller, N., Devaney, A., McNeill, R. E., Davoren, P. A., Lemetre, C., … Kerin, M. J. (2009). MicroRNA signatures predict oestrogen receptor, progesterone receptor and HER2/neu receptor status in breast cancer. *Breast Cancer Research*, *11*(3), R27. http://dx.doi.org/10.1186/bcr2257. bcr2257 [pii].

Lund, M. J., Trivers, K. F., Porter, P. L., Coates, R. J., Leyland-Jones, B., Brawley, O. W., … Eley, J. W. (2009). Race and triple negative threats to breast cancer survival: A population-based study in Atlanta, GA. *Breast Cancer Research and Treatment*, *113*(2), 357–370. http://dx.doi.org/10.1007/s10549-008-9926-3.

Maes, O. C., An, J., Sarojini, H., Wu, H., & Wang, E. (2008). Changes in MicroRNA expression patterns in human fibroblasts after low-LET radiation. *Journal of Cellular Biochemistry*, *105*(3), 824–834. http://dx.doi.org/10.1002/jcb.21878.

Martin, D. N., Boersma, B. J., Yi, M., Reimers, M., Howe, T. M., Yfantis, H. G., … Ambs, S. (2009). Differences in the tumor microenvironment between African-American and European-American breast cancer patients. *PLoS One*, *4*(2), e4531. http://dx.doi.org/10.1371/journal.pone.0004531.

Matamala, N., Vargas, M. T., Gonzalez-Campora, R., Minambres, R., Arias, J. I., Menendez, P., … Benitez, J. (2015). Tumor microRNA expression profiling identifies circulating microRNAs for early breast cancer detection. *Clinical Chemistry*, *61*(8), 1098–1106. http://dx.doi.org/10.1373/clinchem.2015.238691. clinchem.2015. 238691 [pii].

Mbonde, M. P., Amir, H., Akslen, L. A., & Kitinya, J. N. (2001). Expression of oestrogen and progesterone receptors, Ki-67, p53 and BCL-2 proteins, cathepsin D, urokinase plasminogen activator and urokinase plasminogen activator-receptors in carcinomas of the female breast in an African population. *East African Medical Journal*, *78*(7), 360–365.

Mittelbrunn, M., Gutierrez-Vazquez, C., Villarroya-Beltri, C., Gonzalez, S., Sanchez-Cabo, F., Gonzalez, M. A., … Sanchez-Madrid, F. (2011). Unidirectional transfer of microRNA-loaded exosomes from T cells to antigen-presenting cells. *Nature Communications*, *2*, 282. http://dx.doi.org/10.1038/ncomms1285. ncomms1285 [pii].

Mohammadi-Yeganeh, S., Paryan, M., Arefian, E., Vasei, M., Ghanbarian, H., Mahdian, R., … Soleimani, M. (2016). MicroRNA-340 inhibits the migration, invasion, and metastasis of breast cancer cells by targeting Wnt pathway. *Tumour Biology*, *37*(7), 8993–9000. http://dx.doi.org/10.1007/s13277-015-4513-9. 10.1007/s13277-015-4513-9 [pii].

Mukhtar, R. A., Moore, A. P., Nseyo, O., Baehner, F. L., Au, A., Moore, D. H., … Esserman, L. J. (2011). Elevated PCNA+ tumor-associated macrophages in breast cancer are associated with early recurrence and non-Caucasian ethnicity. *Breast Cancer Research and Treatment*, *130*(2), 635–644. http://dx.doi.org/10.1007/s10549-011-1646-4.

Nandy, S. B., Subramani, R., Rajamanickam, V., Lopez-Valdez, R., Arumugam, A., Boopalan, T., & Lakshmanaswamy, R. (2014). microRNA alterations in ALDH positive mammary epithelial cells: A crucial contributing factor towards breast cancer risk reduction in case of early pregnancy. *BMC Cancer*, *14*, 644. http://dx.doi.org/10.1186/1471-2407-14-644. 1471-2407-14-644 [pii].

Nelson, K. M., & Weiss, G. J. (2008). MicroRNAs and cancer: Past, present, and potential future. *Molecular Cancer Therapeutics*, 7(12), 3655–3660. http://dx.doi.org/10.1158/1535-7163.MCT-08-0586. 7/12/3655 [pii].

Nordentoft, I., Birkenkamp-Demtroder, K., Agerbaek, M., Theodorescu, D., Ostenfeld, M. S., Hartmann, A., … Dyrskjot, L. (2012). miRNAs associated with chemo-sensitivity in cell lines and in advanced bladder cancer. *BMC Medical Genomics*, *5*, 40. http://dx.doi.org/10.1186/1755-8794-5-40. 1755-8794-5-40 [pii].

Paik, S., Tang, G., Shak, S., Kim, C., Baker, J., Kim, W., ... Wolmark, N. (2006). Gene expression and benefit of chemotherapy in women with node-negative, estrogen receptor-positive breast cancer. *Journal of Clinical Oncology*, *24*(23), 3726–3734. http://dx.doi.org/10.1200/JCO.2005.04.7985. JCO.2005.04.7985 [pii].

Qiao, A., Gu, F., Guo, X., Zhang, X., & Fu, L. (2016). Breast cancer-associated fibroblasts: Their roles in tumor initiation, progression and clinical applications. *Frontiers of Medicine*, *10*(1), 33–40. http://dx.doi.org/10.1007/s11684-016-0431-5. 10.1007/s11684-016-0431-5 [pii].

Qu, H., Zheng, L., Pu, J., Mei, H., Xiang, X., Zhao, X., ... Tong, Q. (2015). miRNA-558 promotes tumorigenesis and aggressiveness of neuroblastoma cells through activating the transcription of heparanase. *Human Molecular Genetics*, *24*(9), 2539–2551. http://dx.doi.org/10.1093/hmg/ddv018. ddv018 [pii].

Rummel, S., Penatzer, C. E., Shriver, C. D., & Ellsworth, R. E. (2014). PSPHL and breast cancer in African American women: Causative gene or population stratification? *BMC Genetics*, *15*, 38. http://dx.doi.org/10.1186/1471-2156-15-38. 1471-2156-15-38 [pii].

Sakurai, M., Miki, Y., Masuda, M., Hata, S., Shibahara, Y., Hirakawa, H., ... Sasano, H. (2012). LIN28: A regulator of tumor-suppressing activity of let-7 microRNA in human breast cancer. *The Journal of Steroid Biochemistry and Molecular Biology*, *131*(3–5), 101–106. http://dx.doi.org/10.1016/j.jsbmb.2011.10.007. S0960-0760(11)00217-2 [pii].

Schultz, N. A., Andersen, K. K., Roslind, A., Willenbrock, H., Wojdemann, M., & Johansen, J. S. (2012). Prognostic microRNAs in cancer tissue from patients operated for pancreatic cancer—Five microRNAs in a prognostic index. *World Journal of Surgery*, *36*(11), 2699–2707. http://dx.doi.org/10.1007/s00268-012-1705-y.

Sempere, L. F., Christensen, M., Silahtaroglu, A., Bak, M., Heath, C. V., Schwartz, G., ... Cole, C. N. (2007). Altered MicroRNA expression confined to specific epithelial cell subpopulations in breast cancer. *Cancer Research*, *67*(24), 11612–11620. http://dx.doi.org/10.1158/0008-5472.CAN-07-5019. 67/24/11612 [pii].

Shohet, J. M., Ghosh, R., Coarfa, C., Ludwig, A., Benham, A. L., Chen, Z., ... Gunaratne, P. H. (2011). A genome-wide search for promoters that respond to increased MYCN reveals both new oncogenic and tumor suppressor microRNAs associated with aggressive neuroblastoma. *Cancer Research*, *71*(11), 3841–3851. http://dx.doi.org/10.1158/0008-5472.CAN-10-4391. 0008-5472.CAN-10-4391 [pii].

Siegel, R. L., Miller, K. D., & Jemal, A. (2015). Cancer statistics, 2015. *CA: A Cancer Journal for Clinicians*, *65*(1), 5–29. http://dx.doi.org/10.3322/caac.21254.

Siegel, R., Ward, E., Brawley, O., & Jemal, A. (2011). Cancer statistics, 2011: The impact of eliminating socioeconomic and racial disparities on premature cancer deaths. *CA: a Cancer Journal for Clinicians*, *61*(4), 212–236. http://dx.doi.org/10.3322/caac.20121.

Slaby, O., Svoboda, M., Fabian, P., Smerdova, T., Knoflickova, D., Bednarikova, M., ... Vyzula, R. (2007). Altered expression of miR-21, miR-31, miR-143 and miR-145 is related to clinicopathologic features of colorectal cancer. *Oncology*, *72*(5–6), 397–402. http://dx.doi.org/10.1159/000113489. 000113489 [pii].

Smith, B. D., Jiang, J., McLaughlin, S. S., Hurria, A., Smith, G. L., Giordano, S. H., & Buchholz, T. A. (2011). Improvement in breast cancer outcomes over time: Are older women missing out? *Journal of Clinical Oncology*, *29*(35), 4647–4653. http://dx.doi.org/10.1200/JCO.2011.35.8408.

Sorlie, T., Perou, C. M., Tibshirani, R., Aas, T., Geisler, S., Johnsen, H., ... Borresen-Dale, A. L. (2001). Gene expression patterns of breast carcinomas distinguish tumor subclasses with clinical implications. *Proceedings of the National Academy of Sciences of the United States of America*, *98*(19), 10869–10874. http://dx.doi.org/10.1073/pnas.191367098. 98/19/10869 [pii].

Su, B., Zhao, W., Shi, B., Zhang, Z., Yu, X., Xie, F., ... Zhou, L. (2014). Let-7d suppresses growth, metastasis, and tumor macrophage infiltration in renal cell carcinoma by targeting COL3A1 and CCL7. *Molecular Cancer*, *13*, 206. http://dx.doi.org/10.1186/1476-4598-13-206. 1476-4598-13-206 [pii].

Sukata, T., Sumida, K., Kushida, M., Ogata, K., Miyata, K., Yabushita, S., & Uwagawa, S. (2011). Circulating microRNAs, possible indicators of progress of rat hepatocarcinogenesis from early stages. *Toxicology Letters*, *200*(1–2), 46–52. http://dx.doi.org/10.1016/j.toxlet.2010.10.013. S0378-4274(10)01738-8 [pii].

Tambe, M., Pruikkonen, S., Maki-Jouppila, J., Chen, P., Elgaaen, B. V., Straume, A. H., … Kallio, M. J. (2016). Novel Mad2-targeting miR-493-3p controls mitotic fidelity and cancer cells' sensitivity to paclitaxel. *Oncotarget*, 7(11), 12267–12285. http://dx.doi.org/10.18632/oncotarget.7860.

Tanaka, T., Arai, M., Jiang, X., Sugaya, S., Kanda, T., Fujii, K., … Yokosuka, O. (2014). Downregulation of microRNA-431 by human interferon-beta inhibits viability of medulloblastoma and glioblastoma cells via upregulation of SOCS6. *International Journal of Oncology*, *44*(5), 1685–1690. http://dx.doi.org/10.3892/ijo.2014.2317.

Tanic, M., Yanowski, K., Gomez-Lopez, G., Rodriguez-Pinilla, M. S., Marquez-Rodas, I., Osorio, A., … Benitez, J. (2015). MicroRNA expression signatures for the prediction of BRCA1/2 mutation-associated hereditary breast cancer in paraffin-embedded formalin-fixed breast tumors. *International Journal of Cancer*, *136*(3), 593–602. http://dx.doi.org/10.1002/ijc.29021.

Tavazoie, S. F., Alarcon, C., Oskarsson, T., Padua, D., Wang, Q., Bos, P. D., … Massague, J. (2008). Endogenous human microRNAs that suppress breast cancer metastasis. *Nature*, *451*(7175), 147–152. http://dx.doi.org/10.1038/nature06487. nature06487 [pii].

Torres-Martin, M., Lassaletta, L., de Campos, J. M., Isla, A., Gavilan, J., Pinto, G. R., … Rey, J. A. (2013). Global profiling in vestibular schwannomas shows critical deregulation of microRNAs and upregulation in those included in chromosomal region 14q32. *PLoS One*, *8*(6), e65868. http://dx.doi.org/10.1371/journal.pone.0065868. PONE-D-13-03425 [pii].

Valadi, H., Ekstrom, K., Bossios, A., Sjostrand, M., Lee, J. J., & Lotvall, J. O. (2007). Exosome-mediated transfer of mRNAs and microRNAs is a novel mechanism of genetic exchange between cells. *Nature Cell Biology*, *9*(6), 654–659. http://dx.doi.org/10.1038/ncb1596. ncb1596 [pii].

Verma, A. M., Patel, M., Aslam, M. I., Jameson, J., Pringle, J. H., Wurm, P., & Singh, B. (2015). Circulating plasma microRNAs as a screening method for detection of colorectal adenomas. *Lancet*, *385*(Suppl. 1), S100. http://dx.doi.org/10.1016/S0140-6736(15)60415-9. S0140-6736(15)60415-9 [pii].

Volinia, S., Calin, G. A., Liu, C. G., Ambs, S., Cimmino, A., Petrocca, F., … Croce, C. M. (2006). A microRNA expression signature of human solid tumors defines cancer gene targets. *Proceedings of the National Academy of Sciences of the United States of America*, *103*(7), 2257–2261. http://dx.doi.org/10.1073/pnas.0510565103. 0510565103 [pii].

Volinia, S., Galasso, M., Sana, M. E., Wise, T. F., Palatini, J., Huebner, K., & Croce, C. M. (2012). Breast cancer signatures for invasiveness and prognosis defined by deep sequencing of microRNA. *Proceedings of the National Academy of Sciences of the United States of America*, *109*(8), 3024–3029. http://dx.doi.org/10.1073/pnas.1200010109. 1200010109 [pii].

Wallace, T. A., Prueitt, R. L., Yi, M., Howe, T. M., Gillespie, J. W., Yfantis, H. G., … Ambs, S. (2008). Tumor immunobiological differences in prostate cancer between African-American and European-American men. *Cancer Research*, *68*(3), 927–936. http://dx.doi.org/10.1158/0008-5472.CAN-07-260868/3/927.

Wang, S., Huang, J., Lyu, H., Lee, C. K., Tan, J., Wang, J., & Liu, B. (2013). Functional cooperation of miR-125a, miR-125b, and miR-205 in entinostat-induced downregulation of erbB2/erbB3 and apoptosis in breast cancer cells. *Cell Death & Disease*, *4*, e556. http://dx.doi.org/10.1038/cddis.2013.79. cddis201379 [pii].

Weng, L., Ziliak, D., Lacroix, B., Geeleher, P., & Huang, R. S. (2014). Integrative "omic" analysis for tamoxifen sensitivity through cell based models. *PLoS One*, *9*(4), e93420. http://dx.doi.org/10.1371/journal.pone.0093420. PONE-D-13-54390 [pii].

Wiemer, E. A. (2007). The role of microRNAs in cancer: No small matter. *European Journal of Cancer*, *43*(10), 1529–1544. http://dx.doi.org/10.1016/j.ejca.2007.04.002. S0959-8049(07)00292-4 [pii].

Willis, B. C., Liebler, J. M., Luby-Phelps, K., Nicholson, A. G., Crandall, E. D., du Bois, R. M., & Borok, Z. (2005). Induction of epithelial–mesenchymal transition in alveolar epithelial cells by transforming growth factor-beta1: Potential role in idiopathic pulmonary fibrosis. *The American Journal of Pathology*, *166*(5), 1321–1332. S0002-9440(10)62351-6 [pii].

Wu, Z. S., Wu, Q., Wang, C. Q., Wang, X. N., Huang, J., Zhao, J. J., … Zhang, N. (2011). miR-340 inhibition of breast cancer cell migration and invasion through targeting of oncoprotein c-Met. *Cancer*, *117*(13), 2842–2852. http://dx.doi.org/10.1002/cncr.25860.

Wu, H., Zhu, S., & Mo, Y. Y. (2009). Suppression of cell growth and invasion by miR-205 in breast cancer. *Cell Research*, *19*(4), 439–448. http://dx.doi.org/10.1038/cr.2009.18. cr200918 [pii].

Yamamoto, Y., Yoshioka, Y., Minoura, K., Takahashi, R. U., Takeshita, F., Taya, T., … Ochiya, T. (2011). An integrative genomic analysis revealed the relevance of microRNA and gene expression for drug-resistance in human breast cancer cells. *Molecular Cancer*, *10*, 135. http://dx.doi.org/10.1186/1476-4598-10-135. 1476-4598-10-135 [pii].

Yan, L. X., Huang, X. F., Shao, Q., Huang, M. Y., Deng, L., Wu, Q. L., … Shao, J. Y. (2008). MicroRNA miR-21 overexpression in human breast cancer is associated with advanced clinical stage, lymph node metastasis and patient poor prognosis. *RNA*, *14*(11), 2348–2360. http://dx.doi.org/10.1261/rna.1034808. rna.1034808 [pii].

Yanaihara, N., Caplen, N., Bowman, E., Seike, M., Kumamoto, K., Yi, M., … Harris, C. C. (2006). Unique microRNA molecular profiles in lung cancer diagnosis and prognosis. *Cancer Cell*, *9*(3), 189–198. http://dx.doi.org/10.1016/j.ccr.2006.01.025. S1535-6108(06)00033-X [pii].

Yao, S. (2016). MicroRNA biogenesis and their functions in regulating stem cell potency and differentiation. *Biological Procedures Online*, *18*, 8. http://dx.doi.org/10.1186/s12575-016-0037-y.

Yao, S., Graham, K., Shen, J., Campbell, L. E., Singh, P., Zirpoli, G., … Zhao, H. (2013). Genetic variants in microRNAs and breast cancer risk in African American and European American women. *Breast Cancer Research and Treatment*, *141*(3), 447–459. http://dx.doi.org/10.1007/s10549-013-2698-4.

Yarney, J., Vanderpuye, V., & Clegg Lamptey, J. N. (2008). Hormone receptor and HER-2 expression in breast cancers among Sub-Saharan African women. *The Breast Journal*, *14*(5), 510–511. http://dx.doi.org/10.1111/j.1524-4741.2008.00636.x. TBJ636 [pii].

Zanette, D. L., Rivadavia, F., Molfetta, G. A., Barbuzano, F. G., Proto-Siqueira, R., Silva-Jr, W. A., … Zago, M. A. (2007). miRNA expression profiles in chronic lymphocytic and acute lymphocytic leukemia. *Brazilian Journal of Medical and Biological Research*, *40*(11), 1435–1440. doi: S0100-879X2007001100003 [pii].

Zeng, C., Wen, W., Morgans, A. K., Pao, W., Shu, X. O., & Zheng, W. (2015). Disparities by race, age, and sex in the improvement of survival for major cancers: Results from the National Cancer Institute Surveillance, Epidemiology, and End Results (SEER) Program in the United States, 1990 to 2010. *JAMA Oncology*, *1*(1), 88–96. http://dx.doi.org/10.1001/jamaoncol.2014.161.

Zhang, L., Huang, J., Yang, N., Greshock, J., Megraw, M. S., Giannakakis, A., … Coukos, G. (2006). microRNAs exhibit high frequency genomic alterations in human cancer. *Proceedings of the National Academy of Sciences of the United States of America, 103*(24), 9136–9141. http://dx.doi.org/10.1073/pnas.0508889103. 0508889103 [pii].

Zhao, H., Shen, J., Medico, L., Wang, D., Ambrosone, C. B., & Liu, S. (2010). A pilot study of circulating miRNAs as potential biomarkers of early stage breast cancer. *PLoS One, 5*(10), e13735. http://dx.doi.org/10.1371/journal.pone.0013735.

Zheng, H., Zhang, L., Zhao, Y., Yang, D., Song, F., Wen, Y., … Chen, K. (2013). Plasma miRNAs as diagnostic and prognostic biomarkers for ovarian cancer. *PLoS One, 8*(11), e77853. http://dx.doi.org/10.1371/journal.pone.0077853. PONE-D-13-25782 [pii].

Zhu, S., Si, M. L., Wu, H., & Mo, Y. Y. (2007). MicroRNA-21 targets the tumor suppressor gene tropomyosin 1 (TPM1). *The Journal of Biological Chemistry, 282*(19), 14328–14336. http://dx.doi.org/10.1074/jbc.M611393200. M611393200 [pii].

Zhu, S., Wu, H., Wu, F., Nie, D., Sheng, S., & Mo, Y. Y. (2008). MicroRNA-21 targets tumor suppressor genes in invasion and metastasis. *Cell Research, 18*(3), 350–359. http://dx.doi.org/10.1038/cr.2008.24. cr200824 [pii].

CHAPTER FOUR

# Applying a Conceptual Framework to Maximize the Participation of Diverse Populations in Cancer Clinical Trials

**A. Napoles*, E. Cook†, T. Ginossar‡, K.D. Knight§, M.E. Ford¶,1**

*University of California, San Francisco, CA, United States
†University of Texas MD Anderson Cancer Center, Houston, TX, United States
‡University of New Mexico, Albuquerque, NM, United States
§Medical University of South Carolina, Charleston, SC, United States
¶Hollings Cancer Center, Medical University of South Carolina, Charleston, SC, United States
[1]Corresponding author: e-mail address: fordmar@musc.edu

## Contents



## Abstract

The underrepresentation of ethnically diverse populations in cancer clinical trials results in the inequitable distribution of the risks and benefits of this research. Using a case study approach, we apply a conceptual framework of factors associated with the participation of diverse population groups in cancer clinical trials developed by Dr. Jean Ford and colleagues to increase understanding of the specific strategies, and barriers and promoters addressed by these strategies, that resulted in marked success in accrual of racially and ethnically diverse populations in cancer clinical research. Results indicate that the studies presented were able to successfully engage minority participants due to the creation and implementation of multilevel, multifaceted strategies that included: culturally and linguistically appropriate outreach, education, and research studies that were accessible in local communities; infrastructure to support engagement of key stakeholders, clinicians, and organizations serving minority communities; testimonials by ethnically diverse cancer survivors; availability of medical interpretation services;

*Advances in Cancer Research*, Volume 133
ISSN 0065-230X
http://dx.doi.org/10.1016/bs.acr.2016.08.004

and providing infrastructure that facilitated the engagement in clinical research of clinicians who care for minority patient populations. These strategic efforts were effective in addressing limited awareness of trials, lack of opportunities to participate, and acceptance of engagement in cancer clinical trials. Careful attention to the context and population characteristics in which cancer clinical trials are conducted will be necessary to address disparities in research participation and cancer outcomes. These studies illustrate that progress on minority accrual into clinical research requires intentional efforts to overcome barriers at all three stages of the accrual process: awareness, opportunity, and acceptance of participation.

## 1. INTRODUCTION

Cancer is a major public health problem, with racial and ethnic minorities bearing a disproportionate burden of cancer morbidity and mortality relative to other groups. Despite their disproportionate burden of cancer, racial and ethnic minorities are less likely to participate in cancer clinical trials (Ford, Howerton, Lai, et al., 2008; Ford, Siminoff, Pickelsimer, et al., 2013; Ford et al., 2012; Langford, Resnicow, & Lawrence, 2010; Seifer, Michaels, & Collins, 2010). The underrepresentation of ethnically diverse populations in cancer clinical trials results in the inequitable distribution of the risks and benefits of this research (Hartz et al., 2011). The National Institute of Health (NIH) Revitalization Act stipulates that investigators make every effort to achieve participation rates among racial and ethnic minorities that mirror their representation in the US population or in the geographic regions where the trials take place (Pinsky et al., 2008). However, in 2013, only 2% of National Cancer Institute (NCI) sponsored clinical trials focused on racial/ethnic minorities, a proportion substantially lower than their percentage of the US population (36.3%) (Chen, Lara, Dang, Paterniti, & Kelly, 2014).

Using a conceptual framework of factors that can affect the degree of success in recruiting and retaining ethnically diverse populations in research can facilitate and inform the development of strategies to address disparities in clinical research participation. Jean Ford and colleagues (Ford et al., 2008) developed such a framework. Their model describes two categories of factors that can affect accrual during distinct and consecutive phases of the recruitment process: (1) awareness barriers/promoters and (2) acceptance or refusal barriers/promoters. In addition, the model specifies two general types of moderators that can affect the utility of various recruitment strategies used

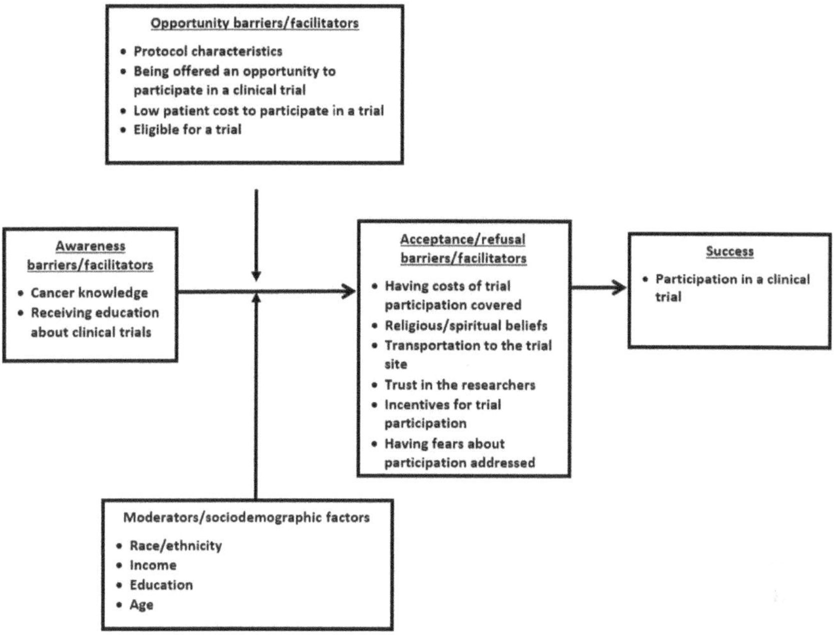


**Fig. 1** Conceptual framework.

throughout the phases (Fig. 1): sociodemographic factors and opportunity barriers/promoters (Ford et al., 2008). In this paper, we utilize the framework as a valuable heuristic for understanding the types of factors that affected recruitment in three studies that included ethnically diverse populations across different population groups and contexts. Therefore, the elements of the Jean Ford et al. (Ford et al., 2008) framework are presented from the perspective of clinical trial participation barriers.

## 2. METHODS

We employ a case study approach to illustrate how the Ford framework can be used to increase our understanding of factors that impede or promote research participation among diverse populations and develop recruitment plans that take into account these factors. First, we describe briefly each stage of the Ford model and its implications for equitable enrollment of racial and ethnic minorities in clinical research. Then, we present three case studies in which we apply the model to understand the effectiveness of specific strategies, to identify potential challenges and successful strategies for engaging ethnically diverse populations in cancer clinical trials based on our experiences and the framework.

## 2.1 Clinical Trial Participation Barriers Identified in the Conceptual Framework

In the Jean Ford et al. (Ford et al., 2008) conceptual framework, awareness barriers refer factors contributing to lack of awareness that trials are open and accruing. Opportunity barriers refer to lack of a personal invitation to participate in a trial, as well as lack of trial access. Acceptance barriers refer to a lack of strategies to address factors that could lead individuals to refuse clinical trial participation, even when offered. These factors include perceptions of the health-care settings where trials are conducted, cancer risk perceptions, and health beliefs.

### 2.1.1 *Awareness Barriers*

Based on the model, awareness barriers can include limited information about cancer and lack of awareness or knowledge of clinical trials (Green et al., 2015; Haynes-Maslow et al., 2014; Leiter, Diefenbach, Doucette, Oh, & Galsky, 2015). These factors could be major contributors to lower participation rates in cancer clinical trials among racially and ethnically diverse populations. Lack of awareness of clinical trials is common among diverse populations with low educational attainment, including African Americans and Asians, and is associated with negative perceptions of trial participation (Advani et al., 2003; Ford et al., 2013; Lara et al., 2005). Awareness barriers to clinical trial participation include lack of culturally appropriate information regarding the importance of research on cancer treatments or behavioral interventions and limited cancer knowledge.

### 2.1.2 *Opportunity Barriers*

In the Ford conceptual framework (Ford et al., 2008), a major factor influencing study participation is having an opportunity to participate in a cancer clinical trial. Thus, providing ethnic minorities with access to cancer clinical trials is a promising approach to address disparities in participation. Factors that promote opportunity to participate in cancer clinical trials include physicians' knowledge and presentation of opportunities for participating in clinical trials to patients. However, studies have shown that physicians may be unaware that their ethnic minority patients may require additional information related to the importance of participation in clinical trials (Ford et al., 2013; Langford et al., 2010). Whether physicians inform their patients of an open clinical trial depends on several factors, including their knowledge of the trial, beliefs about the trial, and beliefs about whether their patients can successfully enroll and complete the trial (Fouad, Reed, & Martin, 2011).

In addition to physician referrals, the setting in which a clinical trial takes place affects the opportunity to participate. For example, patients' geographic distance to the clinical trial location may serve as a serious impediment to participation, especially among low income and ethnically diverse patients who tend to be more likely to experience transportation issues (Brown, Fouad, Basen-Engquist, & Tortolero-Luna, 2000; Wallace & Bartlett, 2013; Williams et al., 2011). Distance from a physician's practice to the nearest clinical trial site was inversely associated with physician referral to and patient enrollment in a trial (Kaplan et al., 2013) suggesting that geographic distance is an important determinant of clinical trial participation.

### 2.1.3 Acceptance Barriers

Acceptance barriers are addressed when patients are educated about cancer clinical trials and given a meaningful opportunity to participate. Under these conditions, it is anticipated that disparities in cancer clinical trial participation rates could be greatly diminished. In fact, a metaanalysis of 20 health research studies reporting on the enrollment decisions of over 70,000 individuals found that when access to studies was provided, participation rates of ethnic minorities and whites did not differ significantly, and in clinical intervention studies, rates were actually higher for Latinos than whites or African Americans (Wendler et al., 2006). Perceptions of the health-care settings where the trial takes place can influence the decision to accept an invitation to participate (Ford et al., 2013; Fouad et al., 2011). For example, if a health-care setting historically provided a segregated system of health care prior to integration, lingering negative perceptions of it may exist in local communities of color. Also, if a health-care system is viewed by community members as not being responsive to the needs or concerns of local diverse communities, this perception could negatively affect community members' views of the clinical staff and/or investigators in the system who conducts clinical trials. Other factors include the cultural and linguistic competence of trials. A study of multilevel factors associated with participation among ethnically diverse women in 230 breast cancer clinical trials found that the provision of study information in English-only and the lack of community outreach were common and significant barriers to the enrollment of ethnic minorities (Livaudais-Toman, Burke, Napoles, & Kaplan, 2014).

Other factors that influence acceptance of participation in cancer clinical trials include risk perceptions and health beliefs. According to the Health Belief Model, increased perceived risk of a potential diagnosis (or perception of recurrence risk) is associated with behavior change to reduce that risk (Glanz, Lewis, & Rimer, 1997; Janz & Becker, 1984; Lipkus, Iden, Terrenoire, & Feaganes, 1999). Thus, providing ethnic minorities with information on their higher risk of poorer quality cancer care and outcomes relative to whites could serve to promote acceptance of participation in cancer clinical trials. Alternatively, however, this information could also play a role in reducing trust in the researchers conducting the trials.

#### *2.1.4 Moderators of Participation in Clinical Trials: Sociodemographic Characteristics*

Sociodemographic factors such as age, income, and education also play a role; individuals who participate in cancer research are more likely to be better educated and to have higher income levels than nonparticipants (Bernard-Davila et al., 2015; Bussey-Jones et al., 2010; Kehl et al., 2014; Unger, Gralow, Albain, Ramsey, & Hershman, 2016). Furthermore, individuals with these characteristics have a higher likelihood of being offered opportunities to participate in cancer research compared with individuals who are less well educated and who have lower income levels (Bernard-Davila et al., 2015; Kehl et al., 2014; Unger et al., 2016). Hence, individuals of a higher socioeconomic status may be more aware of cancer research, have more opportunities to participate, and face fewer economic and logistical barriers to participation than less educated and lower income individuals.

## 3. RESULTS

### 3.1 Case Studies of the Application of the Conceptual Framework

Next, we present case studies in which we applied the conceptual framework to understand the factors that influenced successful enrollment of ethnic minorities in three clinical trials. For each study, we present the study design and accrual results, application of the conceptual framework, and a summary of major highlights.

### *3.1.1 Case Study 1: The Selenium and Vitamin E Cancer Prevention Trial (SELECT)*

#### 3.1.1.1 Study Design and Results

SELECT was a phase III study assessing the impact of selenium and vitamin E, alone and in combination, on the incidence of prostate cancer. SELECT was designed as a double blind, placebo-controlled, two-by-two factorial trial with planned accrual of 32,400 men. The accrual period was designed to last 5 years with a follow-up period of 7–12 years depending on when the participant entered the trial. Men were recruited from over 400 SELECT study sites in the United States, Canada, and Puerto Rico. The minority recruitment goals for SELECT were 20% African Americans, 3% Latinos, and 1% Asians. Black men were oversampled because of their higher prostate cancer incidence and mortality rates.

Fifteen percent of participants accrued to the SELECT trial were African American (vs the targeted goal of 20%), representing the highest percentage of blacks ever recruited to a cancer prevention trial. Because of the successful overall recruitment strategies employed, SELECT closed accrual more than 2 years early, with a total of 35,333 men recruited, exceeding the targeted goal of 32,400. Latinos comprised 6% of the sample vs a goal of 3%, and Asian American accrual was on target at 1%. Minority recruitment to SELECT is described in detail by Cook et al. (2005).

#### 3.1.1.2 Application of the Conceptual Framework

**3.1.1.2.1 Awareness Barriers/Promoters** Patient level promoters included the development of African American sensitive videos and patient education materials, and targeted community outreach activities. For example, "For Men Only" retreats, men's health education sessions across the country that included clinical trial and SELECT information conducted in collaboration with the National Black Leadership Initiative on Cancer III (NBLIC III) were important in spreading the work about the trial. The "Wellness on Wheels" initiative was a similar education program conducted on trains that were frequented by African American men. Two faith-based programs, "Taking it to the Top" and "SELECT Sunday," also had local SELECT site participation. SELECT sites partnered with churches and mosques where pastors delivered the prostate cancer and SELECT message from the pulpit. Prostate cancer survivors were often present and served as advocates for the SELECT trial, giving testimonials about the study. We also presented SELECT at national and local fraternity meetings that targeted African American men. Extensive outreach was negotiated for no cost radio media tours, a television program, and SELECT information on various websites to enhance awareness of the trial. Provider and system level promoters include presenting SELECT at national physician meetings, including the National Medical Association, Southwest Oncology Group (SWOG), and local physician meetings.

**3.1.1.2.2 Opportunity Barriers/Promoters** Patient level opportunity promoters included allowing men to participate with comorbid conditions, as long as they were controlled, and reducing the minimum age criterion for African American men from 55 to 50 due to the equivalent risk of prostate cancer to white men in that age range. Relaxing eligibility criteria related to comorbidity and age are critical for minority populations because they are more likely to have other chronic illnesses and may be more susceptible at earlier ages (Mathioudakis et al., 2016; Prasad, Helder, Brown, & Schaff, 2016; Yoo, De, Wilkins, Smith, & Blumenthal, 2016). We also provided small site grants each year to assist with retention items, parking, and refreshments. Many of the required SELECT preenrollment participant educational sessions were conducted after working hours.

At the provider and system levels, we encouraged physicians to enroll men in the trial with controlled comorbid conditions. We provided accrual updates by sites to physicians and staff at each semiannual SWOG meeting in hopes of increasing accrual. We conducted three separate 1-day workshops that included discussing recruitment issues/needs, developing mentoring relationships, and sharing recruitment strategies. One workshop included panel discussions with local community leaders and SELECT investigators. Another workshop involved pairing underperforming sites with sites performing well serving as mentors. Workshop proceedings were disseminated to all SELECT staff at the semiannual SWOG/SELECT meetings.

**3.1.1.2.3 Acceptance Barriers/Promoters** SELECT promoted acceptance at the patient level by collaborating with trusted national media personalities and obtaining endorsements by members of well-known community organizations, pastors, and local prostate cancer survivors for many local outreach programs. To promote acceptance at the provider/system levels, SELECT formed the SELECT Minority and Medically Underserved Subcommittee (MMUS) that partnered with the National Black Leadership Initiative on Cancer (NBLIC III) and the American Cancer Society. MMUS had a diverse membership with longstanding relationships in minority communities and minority recruitment expertise. MMUS also monitored overall and African American recruitment with monthly accrual reports listed by site. Further analyses, recommendations, and occasional mentoring were provided to specific sites based on these reports. SELECT awarded Minority Recruitment Enhancement Grants (MREGs) were awarded via a competitive review process to sites that demonstrated the ability to recruit substantial numbers of minorities (Cook et al., 2010). Fifteen sites were awarded grants for 1 or 2 years. Sites were required to provide monthly reports detailing implemented recruitment strategies with a simple success rating per strategy. MREGs often supported additional recruitment and adherence materials and local site staff.

#### 3.1.1.3 Summary

Most of the SELECT recruitment initiatives addressed minority accrual barriers at all three phases of the recruitment process: awareness, opportunity, and acceptance. Strategies that worked well included adjusting eligibility criteria, radio media tours, hiring additional staff, mass mailings, and supporting participants with parking reimbursements, transportation, etc. What rarely or did not work included the television program (SELECT was not mentioned), health fairs, churches, barbershops, laundromats, and networking with clinics and community leaders.

### *3.1.2 Case Study 2: Statewide Cancer Clinical Trial Educational Intervention in South Carolina*

#### 3.1.2.1 Study Design and Results

The "Improving Perceptions of Cancer Clinical Trials" study was designed to address the hypothesis that increasing knowledge about cancer clinical trials leads to more positive perceptions of trials among study participants. Therefore, the study intervention, a cancer clinical trial education program, was conducted with predominantly African American communities in South Carolina. These communities experience large cancer disparities, limited access to quality cancer care, and constitute a large population of African Americans who could potentially gain much from participating in cancer clinical trials. The clinical trial education intervention was part of a larger 4-h evidence-based cancer education program that included a 3-h general cancer information component, a 30-min prostate cancer knowledge component, and a 30-min cancer clinical trials component. The intervention was designed to be highly interactive and "hands on" rather than merely didactic. Participants engaged in role playing and small group activities as they practiced sharing the information that they learned with others.

The intervention took place at 10 sites in 11 counties representing several different geographic regions of South Carolina. These 11 counties (and sites) include Berkeley (Varnertown Indian Community), Georgetown (Georgetown), Charleston (Charleston and Johns Island), Greenville (Greenville), Orangeburg (both Orangeburg sites), Richland (Columbia), Bamberg (Denmark), Florence (Florence), Darlington (Darlington), Hampton (Yemassee), and Williamsburg (Kingstree). The study included a convenience sample of participants residing in counties with large racial disparities in cancer mortality.

A pretest/posttest design was used. The survey instrument assessed general sociodemographic information (e.g., age, race, and income). Perceptions of randomized trials were evaluated using the 7-item Attitudes to Randomized Trial Questionnaire (ARTQ) (Fallowfield et al., 1998). The instrument was interviewer-administered and each question was read aloud to the participants to address health literacy issues. Explanations were provided when participants indicated that statements were unclear to them. The ARTQ includes three domains: positive or negative perceptions of medical research in general, willingness to personally participate in research, and willingness to personally participate in research involving randomization. Previous validation in mainly European populations showed that ARTQ scores predicted trial enrollment with 80.4% accuracy (Fallowfield et al., 1998).

Of 315 study participants, most were African American (81.4%) and female (84.8%). Slightly more than 60% of participants had at least a college degree. With the exception of one of seven items on the ARTQ, the majority of participants who had less favorable perceptions of cancer clinical trials before the intervention changed their perceptions to more positive ones from pretest to posttest ($p < 0.01$). The exception, item 3, read "usually the only scientific way to compare one treatment with another is for the choice between the two to be made randomly, rather like tossing a coin." When asked about their responses to this item, participants typically stated that their preference was to be assigned to the intervention group, rather than be randomized.

#### 3.1.2.2 Application of the Conceptual Framework

**3.1.2.2.1 Awareness Barriers/Promoters** The intervention focused on awareness promoters and sought to address these in a comprehensive manner. The intervention was designed to promote awareness and ultimately acceptance by helping individuals understand what a cancer clinical trial is, its purpose, and their rights as study participants. All of these factors were addressed in the intervention. It is important to note that given the responses to item 3 of the ARTQ, additional attention could be paid to the discussion of randomization procedures during future cancer clinical trial education interventions.

**3.1.2.2.2 Opportunity Barriers/Promoters** Although the study did not directly target the creation of opportunities for engagement in research, participants were armed with the knowledge and skills to request information from clinicians and other sources regarding the availability of clinical trials.

**3.1.2.2.3 Acceptance Barriers/Promoters** Pre–post intervention results supported that participants' willingness to personally participate in research improved significantly as a result of the educational program. Overall, participants' perceptions of cancer clinical trials were more favorable after the intervention, suggesting that such programs can mitigate barriers to their acceptance.

#### 3.1.2.3 Summary

Study results demonstrate that the intervention positively influenced trial perceptions and willingness to participate in a clinical trial. The intervention was based on the premise that lack of knowledge about trials can lead to negative perceptions of them, which can have a negative impact on trial participation. Recruitment difficulties often arise from misconceptions of what trials are, the randomization process, and participants' rights in the trial. For example, in the present study, the investigators learned that some participants thought that if they were in a cancer clinical trial, they might be given a placebo rather than the treatment that is being tested. The investigators explained that at minimum, participants would receive the current standard of care if they were assigned to the usual care group, and that under no circumstances would patients with cancer receive a placebo, or no treatment at all. This helped to allay their fears. The intervention evolved from Adult Learning Theory (SD, 2003) and Diffusion of Innovation Theory (EM, 2003) in which trained participants then train others and learning is fostered through trusted social networks. The trained study participants have conducted 104 additional cancer clinical trial education sessions in their communities, reaching 3292 people.

To enhance awareness education in future cancer clinical trials, the ARTQ could be administered to potential trial participants to identify those who could benefit from participating in the intervention. Alternatively, the administration of the ARTQ and the intervention could be incorporated as standard recruitment procedures.

### 3.1.3 *Case Study 3: Strategies for Recruitment of Minority Patients to Clinical Trials in an Academic Cancer Center in a Minority–Majority State*

#### 3.1.3.1 Study Design and Results

Effective recruitment of patients to cancer preventative and therapeutic trials in hospitals and clinics that serve large ethnic minority populations has the potential to decrease cancer disparities. This case study reviews strategies employed by a Minority-Serving Academic Cancer Center (MSACC) to increase recruitment of minority patients to clinical trials. The MSACC was funded in 2000 as 1 of 13 centers in the NCI-Funded Minority-Based Community Clinical Oncology Program (MB-CCOP). MB-CCOPs were academic centers in which a minimum of 40% of new cancer cases occurred in minority populations. The minority–majority state with the highest percentage of Latinos and American Indians in the nation was the catchment area for the MSACC and cancer clinical trials. The findings reported here are based on the analysis of qualitative interviews with research administrators and staff in this MSACC and publically available research documents.

The Partnership increased the number of NCI Cooperative Group trials, as well as investigator initiated and industry trials available in the state. Following two funding cycles of 5 years each, the organization developed a network of about 100 physicians, which included all practicing community-based oncologists in the major Metropolitan area and most community-based oncologists in the state. In its first year of operation, the Partnership reported enrolling 76 patients in clinical trials. In the first 5 years, 521 patients were accrued to trials; of these, 319 (61.2%) were ethnic minorities (180 Hispanic, 36 American Indian, and 103 mixed race, other minority, or undeclared). In the following years, they were able to increase accrual drastically and have enrolled nearly 3000 patients in the first decade of operation. Rates of minority patient recruitment remained strong in the following years.

#### 3.1.3.2 Application of the Conceptual Framework

**3.1.3.2.1 Awareness Barriers/Promoters** This Partnership's mission statement included the provision of educational opportunities to raise awareness of clinical trials. Awareness-related strategies included outreach to the general community, conducted by an outreach person contracted by the nonprofit organization Partnership. In addition, two community educators hired by the MSACC targeted Native American and Spanish-speaking communities in the State with information about cancer; however, the amount of attention paid to increasing awareness to cancer clinical trials was limited.

Strategies that were utilized to promote awareness among providers regarding cancer clinical trials consisted of the provision of information about research protocols, research support, and research nurses and staff involved in the administration of cancer clinical trials. Prior to the MSACC and Partnership creation, this type of research support was not available for community physicians who partnered with the MSACC. In interviews, physicians who reported a higher number of patients accrued attributed their engagement to their beliefs in the importance of cancer clinical trials to patients and to science and their training prior to being hired by the MSACC.

**3.1.3.2.2 Opportunity Barriers/Promoters** The MBACC recognized the need to change research infrastructure in order to remove barriers to patient accrual to clinical trials. The MB-CCOP funding allowed the MSACC to recruit new oncology clinical specialists and to develop a new expanded cancer clinical trial infrastructure at the Academic Center and its affiliate sites. The MSACC leadership proactively identified regulatory and administrative barriers to accrual at the MSACC. Practitioners in nonacademic clinical settings in the state were not able to accrue patients to clinical trials citing lack of research staff and knowledge about such trials as barriers. One of the main strategies employed by the MBACC for recruitment of patients to clinical trials included the creation of a nonprofit organization whose mission was to create a statewide Partnership to increase access to clinical trials. The organization, referred to here as the "Partnership," streamlined administrative and regulatory hurdles of accrual, including provision of research staff and Institutional Review Board (IRB) support. As a nonprofit independent legal entity, the Partnership was able to respond efficiently to changes in the regulatory, administrative, and clinical environments.

Opportunity barriers to participation in clinical trials were significant. Patients who were interested in participating in clinical trials had to travel out of state, and the financial, familial, and emotional resources needed for the travel prohibited most patients from participating, particularly those from marginalized communities. Analysis of the interviews revealed that the MBACC and the Partnership leaders focused predominantly on opportunity-related promoters in their strategies to increase recruitment of minority patients to cancer clinical trials. One of the major promoters to patient accrual cited by MBACC and Partnership leaders included the opportunity for patients to access trials in their own communities. Increasing the number of trials available for patients and physicians was achieved by opening trials throughout the state, providing access at different sites, and increasing the number of physicians conducting cancer clinical trials. In addition, these leaders also felt that they were able to increase the number of available CCTs in the state by streamlining the review process by having one Protocol Review and Monitoring Committee that evaluated quality of proposed trials and a centralized IRB that facilitated approval of protocols for all Partnership's sites. Strategies to increase opportunities to participate focused at the provider level, assuming that this strategy when applied in a diverse catchment area would increase opportunities for multiethnic patients to enroll.

At the organizational level, medical translation services at the time of recruitment, mostly in Spanish, served to expand opportunities for the participation of ethnically diverse patients.

**3.1.3.2.3 Acceptance Barriers/Promoters** The MSACC and Partnership relied predominantly on physicians to communicate information and promote acceptance of cancer clinical trials to patients. No communication strategies directly targeted patients with respect to clinical trials accrual. Physicians at the MSACC received support from research staff, including research nurses who participated in screening patients for eligibility and at times also recruited patients.

#### 3.1.3.3 Summary

The case study above demonstrates the importance of increasing opportunity for CCTs participation for minority patients by reducing administrative and clinical barriers to CCTs in minority-serving institutions. Additionally, it underscores the gap in understanding and bridging awareness-related needs among minority patients and the potential for incentivizing academic centers to implement interventions to support CCT-related awareness among minority patients.

## 4. DISCUSSION

Applying the Ford model to the three case studies demonstrates how implementation of strategic promoters to overcome key barriers can increase awareness of clinical research, provide meaningful opportunities to participate, and facilitate informed decisions to participate, thereby contributing to the equitable representation in clinical research of racially and ethnically diverse populations. Key promoters of recruitment and retention of diverse populations included multilevel approaches that targeted patients, physicians, organizations, systems, communities, and an entire state. The use of linguistically and culturally appropriate information and delivery channels was pivotal in increasing awareness. Community-based outreach strategies that engaged key stakeholders from the targeted communities ensured that opportunities to participate and acceptance of research were maximized. Testimonials by ethnically diverse cancer survivors served to enhance acceptance of participation trials. Availability of medical interpretation services was essential in certain geographic areas. And, providing for infrastructure that facilitated the engagement in clinical research of clinicians who care for minority patient populations proved effective.

These studies illustrate that progress on minority accrual into clinical research requires intentional efforts to overcome barriers at all three stages of the accrual process: awareness, opportunity, and acceptance of participation. The case studies highlight the need to take the research to the communities. These studies were able to achieve recruitment and retention targets by implementing systematic approaches that took the research to the minority communities. Such strategies included the placement of educational programs within ethnically diverse communities, building social networks with minority organizations and community providers, and providing research infrastructure and resources within these communities to support engagement in cancer research.

These case studies provide support for the validity of the Ford model. Awareness and acceptance promoters were present when patients were educated about cancer clinical trials and given a meaningful opportunity to participate. These case studies indicate that education that is tailored and taken to communities via outreach can improve attitudes and increase acceptance of clinical research. The Ford model can be elaborated further by addressing sensitizing conditions. For example, preparatory knowledge of the community can enhance recruitment efforts. Formative research with key stakeholders to identify preferred learning styles, social networks, and communication channels can result in more efficient and effective use of recruitment resources.

While a great number of studies have identified barriers to recruitment among racially and ethnically diverse populations, this study serves to illustrate strategies that were applied successfully to enhance participation rates among these populations. However, this success hinged on a culturally informed investment of resources that required key stakeholder input via the establishment of genuine partnerships with the targeted populations and their providers. Most researchers underestimate the time, attention, and resources required to engage minority populations in research (National Academies of Sciences, Engineering, and Medicine, 2016). With the rapid advancement of precision medicine approaches to cancer treatments, issues of genomic literacy, patient distrust and effective clinician–patient communication, as well as equitable access to state-of-the-science treatments, will become even more pronounced. If we continue to dedicate insufficient attention and resources to the engagement of racially and ethnically diverse populations in cancer clinical trials, this could serve to exacerbate disparities in cancer outcomes. Inclusion of these populations in numbers that are proportionate to the populations of persons affected by specific types of cancers is scientifically and ethically sound.

## ACKNOWLEDGMENTS

This research was supported by the following funding sources: NIH/NCI Grant Number P20 CA157071; NIH/NCI Grant Number P30 CA138313; NIH/NIMHD Grant Number R01 MD005892; NIH/NCI Grant Number 3U10CA086780-10S1; ACS IRG Grant Number 92-024; NIH/NCI Grant Number 1U54CA153511; and NIH/NIA Grant Number 1 P30 AG15272.

## REFERENCES

Advani, A. S., Atkeson, B., Brown, C. L., Peterson, B. L., Fish, L., Johnson, J. L., … Gautier, M. (2003). Barriers to the participation of African-American patients with cancer in clinical trials: A pilot study. *Cancer*, *97*(6), 1499–1506.

Bernard-Davila, B., Aycinena, A. C., Richardson, J., Gaffney, A. O., Koch, P., Contento, I., … Greenlee, H. (2015). Barriers and facilitators to recruitment to a culturally-based dietary intervention among urban Hispanic breast cancer survivors. *Journal of Racial and Ethnic Health Disparities*, *2*(2), 244–255. http://dx.doi.org/10.1007/s40615-014-0076-5.

Brown, D. R., Fouad, M. N., Basen-Engquist, K., & Tortolero-Luna, G. (2000). Recruitment and retention of minority women in cancer screening, prevention, and treatment trials. *Annals of Epidemiology*, *10*(8 Suppl.), S13–S21.

Bussey-Jones, J., Garrett, J., Henderson, G., Moloney, M., Blumenthal, C., & Corbie-Smith, G. (2010). The role of race and trust in tissue/blood donation for genetic research. *Genetics in Medicine*, *12*(2), 116–121. http://dx.doi.org/10.1097/GIM.0b013e3181cd6689.

Chen, M. S., Lara, P., Dang, J. H. T., Paterniti, D. A., & Kelly, K. (2014). Twenty years post-NIH revitalization act: Enhancing minority participation in clinical trials (EMPaCT): Laying groundwork for improving minority clinical trial accrual. *Cancer, 120*(7), 1091–1096.

Cook, E. D., Arnold, K. B., Hermos, J. A., McCaskill-Stevens, W., Moody-Thomas, S., Probstfield, J. L., … Minasian, L. M. (2010). Impact of supplemental site grants to increase African American accrual for the Selenium and Vitamin E Cancer Prevention Trial. *Clinical Trials*, 7(1), 90–99. http://dx.doi.org/10.1177/1740774509357227.

Cook, E. D., Moody-Thomas, S., Anderson, K. B., Campbell, R., Hamilton, S. J., Harrington, J. M., … Probstfield, J. L. (2005). Minority recruitment to the Selenium and Vitamin E Cancer Prevention Trial (SELECT). *Clinical Trials, 2*(5), 436–442.

Em, R. (2003). *Diffusion of innovations* (5th ed.). . New York: Free Press.

Fallowfield, L. J., Jenkins, V., Brennan, C., Sawtell, M., Moynihan, C., & Souhami, R. L. (1998). Attitudes of patients to randomised clinical trials of cancer therapy. *European Journal of Cancer, 34*(10), 1554–1559.

Ford, J. G., Howerton, M., Lai, G. Y., et al. (2008). Barriers to recruiting underrepresented population to cancer clinical trials: A systematic review. *Cancer, 112*, 228–242.

Ford, M. E., Siminoff, L., Pickelsimer, E., et al. (2013). Unequal burden of disease, unequal participation in clinical trials: Solutions from African American and Latino community members. *Health & Social Work, 38*, 29–38.

Ford, M., Wahlquist, A., Blake, R., Green, C., Streets, J., Fuller, E., … Garrett-Mayer, E. (2012). Assessing an intervention to improve clinical trial perceptions among predominately African-American communities in South Carolina. *Progress in Community Health Partnerships, 6*(3), 249–263. http://dx.doi.org/10.1353/cpr.2012.0038.

Fouad, M., Reed, D., & Martin, M. (May 2011). *Successful models for minority recruitment [Online Training Course]*. Retrieved from http://www.empactconsortium.com/material/qa-with-dr-jean-ford/#sthash.8lgLTakq.dpuf.

Glanz, K., Lewis, F., & Rimer, B. K. (1997). *Health behavior and health education: Theory, research, and practice*. San Francisco: Jossey-Bass.

Green, M. A., Michaels, M., Blakeney, N., Odulana, A. A., Isler, M. R., Richmond, A., … Corbie-Smith, G. (2015). Evaluating a community-partnered cancer clinical trials pilot intervention with African American communities. *Journal of Cancer Education, 30*(1), 158–166. http://dx.doi.org/10.1007/s13187-014-0764-1.

Hartz, S. M., Johnson, E. O., Saccone, N. L., Hatsukami, D., Breslau, N., & Bierut, L. J. (2011). Inclusion of African Americans in genetic studies: What is the barrier? *American Journal of Epidemiology, 174*(3), 336–344. http://dx.doi.org/10.1093/aje/kwr084.

Haynes-Maslow, L., Godley, P., Dimartino, L., White, B., Odom, J., Richmond, A., & Carpenter, W. (2014). African American women's perceptions of cancer clinical trials. *Cancer Medicine, 3*(5), 1430–1439. http://dx.doi.org/10.1002/cam4.284.

Janz, N. K., & Becker, M. H. (1984). The Health Belief Model: A decade later. *Health Education Quarterly, 11*(1), 1–47. Retrieved from, http://www.ncbi.nlm.nih.gov/pubmed/6392204.

Kaplan, C. P., Napoles, A. M., Dohan, D., Shelley Hwang, E., Melisko, M., Nickleach, D., … Haas, J. (2013). Clinical trial discussion, referral, and recruitment: Physician, patient, and system factors. *Cancer Causes & Control, 24*(5), 979–988. http://dx.doi.org/10.1007/s10552-013-0173-5.

Kehl, K. L., Arora, N. K., Schrag, D., Ayanian, J. Z., Clauser, S. B., Klabunde, C. N., … Keating, N. L. (2014). Discussions about clinical trials among patients with newly diagnosed lung and colorectal cancer. *Journal of the National Cancer Institute, 106*(10), 1–9. http://dx.doi.org/10.1093/jnci/dju216.

Langford, A., Resnicow, K., & Lawrence, A. N. (2010). Clinical trial awareness among racial/ethnic minorities in HINTS 2007: Sociodemographic, attitudinal and knowledge correlates. *Journal of Health Communication: International Perspectives, 15*, 92–101.

Lara, P. N., Jr., Paterniti, D. A., Chiechi, C., Turrell, C., Morain, C., Horan, N., … Chen, M. S., Jr. (2005). Evaluation of factors affecting awareness of and willingness to participate in cancer clinical trials. *Journal of Clinical Oncology, 23*(36), 9282–9289. http://dx.doi.org/10.1200/JCO.2005.02.6245.

Leiter, A., Diefenbach, M. A., Doucette, J., Oh, W. K., & Galsky, M. D. (2015). Clinical trial awareness: Changes over time and sociodemographic disparities. *Clinical Trials, 12*(3), 215–223. http://dx.doi.org/10.1177/1740774515571917.

Lipkus, I. M., Iden, D., Terrenoire, J., & Feaganes, J. R. (1999). Relationships among breast cancer concern, risk perceptions, and interest in genetic testing for breast cancer susceptibility among African-American women with and without a family history of breast cancer. *Cancer Epidemiology, Biomarkers & Prevention, 8*(6), 533–539. Retrieved from, http://www.ncbi.nlm.nih.gov/pubmed/10385144.

Livaudais-Toman, J., Burke, N. J., Napoles, A., & Kaplan, C. P. (2014). Health literate organizations: Are clinical trial sites equipped to recruit minority and limited health literacy patients? *The Journal of Health Disparities Research and Practice*, 7(4), 1–13. Retrieved from, http://www.ncbi.nlm.nih.gov/pubmed/26295011.

Mathioudakis, N. N., Giles, M., Yeh, H. C., Haywood, C., Jr., Greer, R. C., & Golden, S. H. (2016). Racial differences in acute kidney injury of hospitalized adults with diabetes. *Journal of Diabetes and its Complications, 30*(6), 1129–1136. http://dx.doi.org/10.1016/j.jdiacomp.2016.03.031.

National Academies of Sciences, Engineering, and Medicine (2016). *Applying an implementation science approach to genomic medicine.* Washington, DC: Workshop Summary.

Pinsky, P. F., Ford, M., Gamito, E., Higgins, D., Jenkins, V., Lamerato, L., … Gohagan, J. K. (2008). Enrollment of racial and ethnic minorities in the Prostate, Lung, Colorectal and Ovarian Cancer Screening Trial. *Journal of the National Medical Association, 100*(3), 291–298.

Prasad A., Helder M.R., Brown D.A. and Schaff H.V. (2016). Understanding differences in administrative and audited patient data in cardiac: Comparison of the University Health System Consortium and Society of Thoracic Surgeons Databases, *Journal of the American College of Surgeons*, (in press). http://dx.doi.org/10.1016/j.jamcollsurg.2016.06.393.

Sd, B. (2003). Pedagogy and androagogy. In K. R. A. DiStefano, R. Silverman, & S. Taira (Eds.), *Encyclopedia of distributed learning.* Thousand Oaks, CA: Sage.

Seifer, S. D., Michaels, M., & Collins, S. (2010). Applying community-based participatory research principles and approaches in clinical trials: Forging a new model for cancer clinical research. *Progress in Community Health Partnerships, 4*(1), 37–46. http://dx.doi.org/10.1353/cpr.0.0103.

Unger, J. M., Gralow, J. R., Albain, K. S., Ramsey, S. D., & Hershman, D. L. (2016). Patient income level and cancer clinical trial participation: A prospective survey study. *JAMA Oncology, 2*(1), 137–139. http://dx.doi.org/10.1001/jamaoncol.2015.3924.

Wallace, D. C., & Bartlett, R. (2013). Recruitment and retention of African American and Hispanic girls and women in research. *Public Health Nursing, 30*(2), 159–166. http://dx.doi.org/10.1111/phn.12014.

Wendler, D., Kington, R., Madans, J., Van Wye, G., Christ-Schmidt, H., Pratt, L. A., … Emanuel, E. (2006). Are racial and ethnic minorities less willing to participate in health research? *PLoS Medicine, 3*(2), e19. http://dx.doi.org/10.1371/journal.pmed.0030019.

Williams, I. C., Utz, S. W., Jones, R., Hinton, I., Steeves, R., & Alexander, G. (2011). Recruitment of rural African Americans for research projects: Lessons learned. *Southern Online Journal of Nursing Research, 11*(1), 8. Retrieved from, http://www.ncbi.nlm.nih.gov/pubmed/24791157.

Yoo, W., De, S., Wilkins, T., Smith, S. A., & Blumenthal, D. (2016). Age, race and regional disparities in colorectal cancer incidence rates in Georgia between 2000 and 2012. *Annals of Public Health and Research, 3*(2) Retrieved from, http://www.ncbi.nlm.nih.gov/pubmed/27042701.

CHAPTER FIVE

# Social Networks Across Common Cancer Types: The Evidence, Gaps, and Areas of Potential Impact

**L.J. Rice*,[1], C.H. Halbert*,†**

*Hollings Cancer Center, Medical University of South Carolina, Charleston, SC, United States
†Ralph H. Johnson Veterans Affairs Medical Center, Charleston, SC, United States
[1]Corresponding author: e-mail address: ricela@musc.edu

## Contents



## Abstract

Although the association between social context and health has been demonstrated previously, much less is known about network interactions by gender, race/ethnicity, and sociodemographic characteristics. Given the variability in cancer outcomes among groups, research on these relationships may have important implications for addressing cancer health disparities. We examined the literature on social networks and cancer across the cancer continuum among adults. Relevant studies ($N=16$) were identified using two common databases: PubMed and Google Scholar. Most studies used a prospective cohort study design ($n=9$), included women only ($n=11$), and were located in the United States ($n=14$). Seventy-five percent of the studies reviewed used a validated scale or validated items to measure social networks ($n=12$). Only one study examined social network differences by race, 57.1% ($n=8$) focused on breast cancer alone, 14.3% ($n=2$) explored colorectal cancer or multiple cancers simultaneously, and 7.1% ($n=1$) only prostate cancer. More than half of the studies included multiple ethnicities in the

*Advances in Cancer Research*, Volume 133
ISSN 0065-230X
http://dx.doi.org/10.1016/bs.acr.2016.09.002

sample, while one study included only low-income subjects. Despite findings of associations between social networks and cancer survival, risk, and screening, none of the studies utilized social networks as a mechanism for reducing health disparities; however, such an approach has been utilized for infectious disease control. Social networks and the support provided within these networks have important implications for health behaviors and ultimately cancer disparities. This review serves as the first step toward dialog on social networks as a missing component in the social determinants of cancer disparities literature that could move the needle upstream to target adverse cancer outcomes among vulnerable populations.

## 1. INTRODUCTION

Over the last decade, there has been growing interest in understanding the role social context plays in disease development and disproportionate health outcomes (U.S. Department of Health & Human Services [DHHS], 2011). From the establishment of national goals (DHHS, 2011) to studies highlighting associations between social and economic conditions and trends in chronic disease across racial and ethnic lines (Adler & Newman, 2002; Braveman, Cubbin, Egerter, Williams, & Pamuk, 2010; Diderichsen, Evans, & Whitehead, 2001; Williams & Jackson, 2005; Woolf & Braveman, 2011), it is well documented that socially disadvantaged groups are more vulnerable to disease and experience poorer health outcomes than majority groups (Braveman et al., 2010). Though these outcomes exist across disease, the most concerning of health disparities exists in cancer. Cancer is a leading cause of death globally; however, advances across the cancer continuum have led to major reductions in cancer incidence and cancer mortality for many of the common cancers for more than three decades (Kohler et al., 2015; Ryerson et al., 2016). Despite improvements, overall cancer burden inequitably impacts economically disadvantaged persons and racial and ethnic minorities, namely African Americans more than other groups (Siegel, Miller, & Jemal, 2016). Breast cancer mortality rates among African American women are higher than White women who have a higher incidence (Ryerson et al., 2016). African Americans have both higher incidence and mortality rates for the three leading causes of cancer death among men (Ryerson et al., 2016). Furthermore, empirical studies have shown differences across the cancer continuum between African Americans and Whites (Baldwin et al., 2005; Gerend & Pai, 2008; Jepson, Kessler,

Portnoy, & Gibbs, 1991; Li, Malone, & Daling, 2003; Shavers & Brown, 2002). These differences are caused by a complex interplay of biological, social, economic, and environmental factors (Freeman, 2003; Institute of Medicine, 2003).

Underrepresented populations face unique challenges when accessing the health care system. These challenges include no access to a provider or provider shortages, transportation limitations, geographical location, and reduced quality of care (Mead et al., 2008). Compared to Whites, African Americans lack the appropriate resources necessary to manage disease (Davey, Neaton, Wentworth, Stamler, & Stamler, 1998; Evans, Metcalfe, Ibrahim, Persad, & Ben-Shlomo, 2008; Shavers & Brown, 2002; Shavers et al., 2004), and experience longer times between diagnosis and treatment (Kinlock et al., 2016; Stokes et al., 2013; Smith, Ziogas, & Anton-Culver, 2013). Research shows that delays in cancer treatment after diagnosis can lead to a 10% decrease in 5-year breast cancer survival for Hispanics and African Americans (Smith et al., 2013) and decreased survival in prostate cancer among African American men (Kinlock et al., 2016; Stokes et al., 2013; Smith et al., 2013). For all cancer sites combined, men have higher mortality rates than women with a reported 211.6 deaths per 100,000 compared to 147.4 deaths among women (Kohler et al., 2015). In addition, for all cancers, incidence and mortality rates among Black American men exceed those of all other racial or ethnic groups at 587.7 cases and 269.3 deaths per 100,000, respectively (Kohler et al., 2015; Ryerson et al., 2016). Knowing these facts, timely care is critical for survival in this group.

Cancer and its consequences occur within the context of human social environments (Freeman & Chu, 2005). Social environments facilitate or impede resource sharing, reinforce health beliefs as well as health behaviors. Inadequate social environments can have a significant effect on cancer prevention, risk, and survival (Freeman & Chu, 2005). Prior to and after a cancer diagnosis, receiving adequate information to make an informed decision about care and empowering a patient to make an informed decision depends heavily on whether there is access to the appropriate resources including a primary care physician with such knowledge. For example, the American Cancer Society recommends men make an informed decision about prostate cancer screening by learning about the risk, harms, and benefits of screening from their health care provider (Wolf et al., 2010). The underlying assumption is that patients have a primary care physician or access to a reliable source of health information and care. Receiving the appropriate information to make an informed decision can vary by patient. First, because communication between a patient and provider is associated with having a regular healthcare provider, one's age, marital status, as well as other factors including race, annual household income, and having undergone a PSA test (Bhuyan et al., 2015). New evidence from the Health Information National Trends Survey (HINTS) shows minimal discussions occur between patients and providers about PSA testing and prostate cancer treatment options (Bhuyan et al., 2015). Halbert et al. (2015) found that African Americans' decision to ever undergo a PSA test will depend on communication from their provider. Again, the assumption is that health care providers are the primary source of information for patients. A lack of effective or any provider communication, effects patient's informed decision making about screening and ultimately, may lead to misinformation and treatment dissatisfaction (Thomas, Groff, Tsang, & Carlson, 2009), later stage diagnosis, delayed treatment, and decreased survival rates (Song et al., 2014). Understanding the underlying social dynamics between patients and providers, and patients and other social connections may provide more insight into cancer disparities between groups.

Decisions about care, care for early detection, treatment, and prevention are influenced by a network of factors and players (Umberson & Montez, 2010). Identifying these players is important, but of greater importance is determining the impact these "players" and their relationships have on risks and health decisions related to cancer care. The purpose of this review was to examine the evidence on the association between social networks and cancer by gender, socioeconomic status, and race or ethnicity. Emphasis was placed on studies examining common cancers such as breast, lung, and prostate cancer to identify areas for further research in cancer health disparities. Examining social ties' role in cancer care among diverse populations has implications for closing the health disparities gap in many common cancers such as prostate cancer. This chapter will include a brief overview of social networks and health placing emphasis on cancer, the link between in-person and online social networks and cancer, and then highlight differences in social connections by sociodemographic factors. A discussion on the relationship between social factors and lifestyle behaviors, which are important for cancer prevention and control and the normative behaviors that exist within in homophilic networks (networks of similar people), is then provided. Lastly, this chapter addresses the relative usefulness of exploring social networks as a missing component of the social determinants of health approach to promote equity in cancer care and understand barriers to timely care.

## 2. METHODS

A literature review on all studies examining social networks and cancer was performed in March 2016. Two commonly used databases: PubMed and Google Scholar were used to identify relevant articles using the search terms: "social networks" and "cancer." Several studies use "social relationships," "social context," and "social ties" interchangeably when examining social networks. Therefore, we used these terms in our search to identify relevant research on social networks. Initial screening of articles was based on original search terms and their inclusion in a study title and/or abstract. A flow diagram of included and excluded articles is provided in Fig. 1. For inclusion in the review, articles had to be (1) focused on the association between social networks and cancer, (2) published in English, (3) in a peer-reviewed academic journal article or book, and (4) focus on one of four common cancers (breast, prostate, colorectal, and/or lung) among adults. Due to the limited number of articles on the subject matter, all articles that met the inclusion criteria, regardless of publication year, were in the study. The final list of articles are provided in Table 1.

## 3. CANCER, SOCIAL TIES, AND SOCIAL NETWORKS

Berkman, Glass, Brissette, and Seeman's (2000) defines social networks as "the web of social relationships that surround an individual and the characteristics of the ties within those relationships." For the purpose of this review, social networks is operationalized using Berkman et al.'s (2000) conceptual model on how social networks impact health to distinguish between social features that are useful for cancer prevention and control. The association between social relationships and health is well-established empirically (Umberson & Montez, 2010); numerous studies have demonstrated that individuals who are more socially connected or engaged (in social groups or community activities) and have better quality relationships experience better mental and physical health outcomes (Berkman & Glass, 2000; Berkman & Syme, 1979; Blazer, 1982; Cassel, 1976; Cobb, 1976; Cohen, 2004; Cohen & Wills, 1985; Greenblatt, Becerra, & Serafetinides, 1982; House, Landis, & Umberson, 1988; Kawachi & Berkman, 2001; Seeman, 1996; Smith & Christakis, 2008). Studies have linked social connections to many chronic conditions

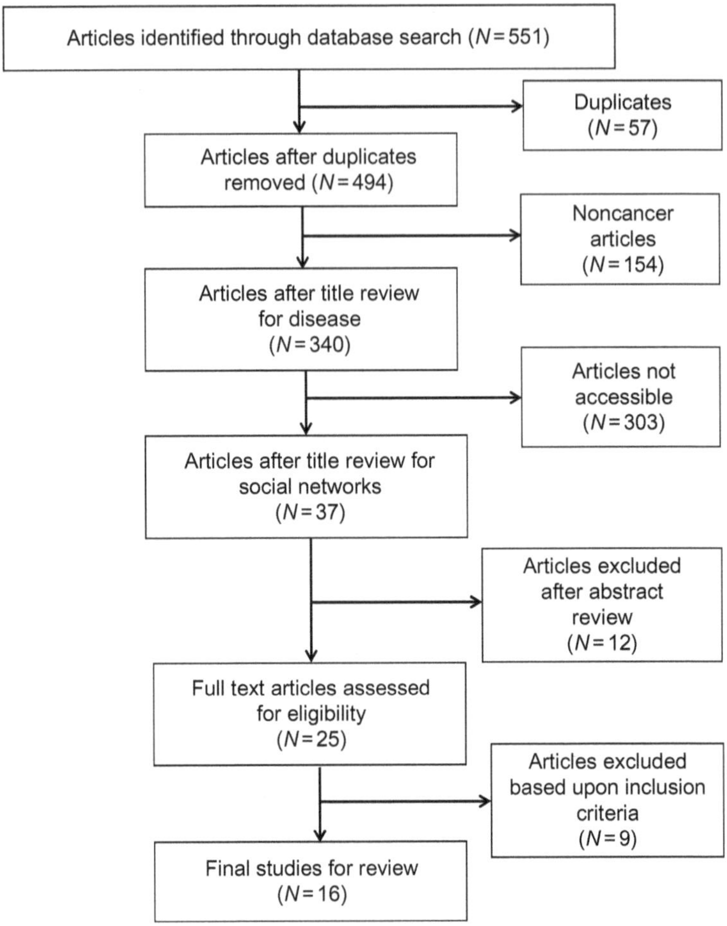


**Fig. 1** Flowchart of social networks articles examined in review.

including cancer (Smith & Christakis, 2008). For example, having few social connections can mean lower survival rates for men (Reynolds & Kaplan, 1990). Social connections have also been linked to cancer risk (Bergelt et al., 2009) and screening behaviors (Suarez et al., 1994), cancer incidence (Reynolds & Kaplan, 1990; Vogt, Mullooly, Ernst, Pope, & Hollis, 1992), cancer mortality (Berkman & Syme, 1979; Kawachi et al., 1996; Orth-Gomer & Johnson, 1987; Pinquart & Duberstein, 2010; Reynolds & Kaplan, 1990; Vogt et al., 1992), cancer survival (Iwasaki et al., 2002; Kroenke et al., 2006; Reynolds et al., 1994), and quality of life (QOL) (Kroenke, Kwan, et al., 2013; Michael et al., 2002). Structural (existence

**Table 1** Studies Examining Social Networks and Cancer

| Study, Author, Year | Study Focus | Cancer Type | Location | Study Type | Social Networks Measure | Participants | | | Demographics | Mean Age, Age Range |
|---|---|---|---|---|---|---|---|---|---|---|
| | | | | | | Total | Male | Female | | |
| Beasley et al. (2010) | How social networks relate to survival after a diagnosis | Breast cancer | USA: New Hampshire, Massachusetts, and Wisconsin | Prospective cohort | Berkman–Syme social network index (SNI) | 4589 | 0 | 4589 | NR | 58.8[b] |
| Bergelt, Prescott, Gronbaek, Koch, and Johansen (2009) | Association between social ties and risk for cancer | Breast cancer, lung cancer, prostate cancer, colorectal cancer | Copenhagen, Denmark | Prospective cohort | Social network score (quantity of social contacts) | 8548 | 3838 | 4710 | NR | 20+ |
| Chamie et al. (2011) | Association between the extent of social support, partnership status, and treatment type | Prostate cancer | USA: California | Prospective cohort | Social support (no scale indicated) | 418 | 418 | 0 | 78 White<br>71 Black<br>239 Hispanic<br>30 Other | 60.7[b] |

*Continued*

**Table 1** Studies Examining Social Networks and Cancer—cont'd

| Study, Author, Year | Study Focus | Cancer Type | Location | Study Type | Social Networks Measure | Participants | | | Demographics | Mean Age, Age Range |
|---|---|---|---|---|---|---|---|---|---|---|
| | | | | | | Total | Male | Female | | |
| Crookes et al. (2016)[a] | Social networks and perceived support for healthy eating | Breast cancer | USA: New York | Randomized–controlled trial | Cohen's SNI; general social Survey social networks module | 34 | 0 | 34 | Latina:<br>10 Black<br>15 White<br>1 Native American<br>2 Mixed race | 56.9 years |
| Kinney, Bloor, Martin, and Sandler (2005) | Relationship between both structural and functional aspects of social ties and utilization of colorectal cancer screening tests | Colorectal cancer | USA: North Carolina | Case–control | SNI | 697 | 353 | 344 | 402 White<br>295 Black | 68 |
| Kroenke, Kubzansky, Schernhammer, Holmes, and Kawachi (2006) | Social ties and survival after breast cancer diagnosis | Breast cancer | USA | Prospective cohort | Berkman–Syme SNI | 2835 | 0 | 2835 | NR | 46–71 years |

| | | | | | | | | | | |
|---|---|---|---|---|---|---|---|---|---|---|
| Kroenke et al. (2012) | Social network members, with mortality outcomes, considering the modifying influence of both social support and social burden | Breast cancer | USA | Observational study | Social network measured using four components | 4530 | 0 | 4530 | Varied by networks size included race/ ethnicity included: Caucasian, African American, Asian, Hispanic/ Latino, Other | 63.8[b] |
| Kroenke, Kwan, et al. (2013) | Mechanisms through which social relationships influence quality of life (QOL) in survivors | Breast cancer | USA: California | Prospective cohort | Berkman–Syme SNI; four components and Arizona activity frequency questionnaire (AAFQ) | 3139 | 0 | 3139 | Varied by networks size included race/ ethnicity included: Caucasian, African American, Asian, Hispanic/ Latino, Other | 59.7[b] |

*Continued*

**Table 1** Studies Examining Social Networks and Cancer—cont'd

| Study, Author, Year | Study Focus | Cancer Type | Location | Study Type | Social Networks Measure | Participants | | | Demographics | Mean Age, Age Range |
|---|---|---|---|---|---|---|---|---|---|---|
| | | | | | | Total | Male | Female | | |
| Kroenke, Quesenberry, et al. (2013) | How levels of social support and burden influence association between larger social networks and lower breast cancer mortality | Breast cancer | USA: California and Utah | Prospective cohort | Social networks; five components | 2264 | 0 | 2264 | Varied by networks size included Race/ Ethnicity included: Caucasian, African American, Asian, Hispanic/ Latino, Other | 58.2[b] |
| Michael, Berkman, Colditz, Holmes, and Kawachi (2002) | Influence of social networks on health-related quality of life (HRQoL) among breast cancer survivors | Breast cancer | USA | Prospective cohort | Modified Berkman–Syme SNI: four levels of connections | 699 | 0 | 699 | NR | 59.1 years; 46–72 years |

| | | | | | | | | | | |
|---|---|---|---|---|---|---|---|---|---|---|
| Reynolds et al. (1994) | Relationship between social ties, stage of disease, and survival | Breast cancer | USA: Georgia, Louisiana, and California | Case–control | Berkman–Syme SNI | 1011 | 0 | 1011 | 525 Black 486 White | 20–79 years |
| Rottenberg et al. (2014) | To assess the association between social networks on survival after cancer diagnosis | Breast, colon, lung, and prostate cancer | Jerusalem, Israel | Historical prospective | Five distinct social networks measured; no scale identified | 3679 | 1758 | 1921 | Ethnic origin: Israel 110 Asia 856 Africa 589 Europe-America 2102 | 72.3 years; 61–101 years |
| Sapp et al. (2003) | Long-term colorectal cancer survivors' health-related quality of life (HRQoL) in relation to social networks | Colorectal cancer | USA: Wisconsin | Prospective cohort | Modified version of the Berkman–Syme SNI | 259 | 0 | 259 | 98% non-Hispanic white, 2% African American/black, one participant was American Indian or Alaskan Native | 72 years (range, 43–84 years) |

*Continued*

**Table 1** Studies Examining Social Networks and Cancer—cont'd

| Study, Author, Year | Study Focus | Cancer Type | Location | Study Type | Social Networks Measure | Participants | | | Demographics | Mean Age, Age Range |
|---|---|---|---|---|---|---|---|---|---|---|
| | | | | | | Total | Male | Female | | |
| Suarez, Lloyd, Weiss, Rainbolt, and Pulley (1994)[c] | The extent to which differences in social networks account for variations in breast and cervical cancer-screening practices among | Breast and cervical cancer | USA: Texas | Cross-sectional | Berkman–Syme SNI; Kang and Bloom; six components | 450 | 0 | 450 | Mexican-American | Aged 40+ |
| Suarez et al. (2000)[c] | Relationship between social networks and cancer screening | Breast and cervical cancer | USA: California | Cross-sectional | Adapted from Berkman–Syme SNI | 2383 | 0 | 2383 | Mexican-American 1550<br>Central American 174<br>Puerto Rican 236<br>Cuban American 279 | Aged 40+ |

| | | | | | | | | | | |
|---|---|---|---|---|---|---|---|---|---|---|
| Ye, Williams, and Xu (2009) | Relationship between social networks and colorectal cancer (CRC) screening among males and females | Colorectal cancer | USA | Prospective cohort | Modified version of Berkman–Syme SNI | 2907 | 960 | 1947 | 83.4% Non-Hispanic White, 4.4 Non-Hispanic Black, 7.4% Hispanic, 4.8% Non-Hispanic Other | 65.5 years; aged 50+ |

[a]Only bivariate associations were examined.
[b]Age was calculated as an average of stratified groups.
[c]Participants include low-income groups.
*NR*, not reported.

and interconnection between members) and functional (perceived support or receipt of resources from networks through interactions) components of social networks are correlated with disease development (Seeman & Syme, 1987), mortality risk (Holt-Lunstad, Smith, & Layton, 2010), and have been shown to predict mortality (House et al., 1988). In a review on social relationships and mortality risk, Holt-Lunstad et al. (2010) found that structural aspects of social networks such as the number of network members, network homogeneity, and frequency of contact amongst members were the strongest predictors of mortality risk. Holt-Lunstad et al. (2010) also found that greater social involvement decreases mortality rates, which corresponds with findings from other studies (Bosworth & Schaie, 1997; House et al., 1988; Seeman, 1996). Robust social relationships, especially those established within communities, have been shown to increase survival rates by as much as 50% regardless of sociodemographics such as age and race (Holt-Lunstad et al., 2010; House et al., 1988).

Social ties, defined by Thoits (2011) as "connections to and contacts with others based upon membership in a primary or secondary group," have been linked to chronic and infectious diseases (Klovdahl et al., 1994). For example, Cohen, Doyle, Skoner, Rabin, and Gwaltney (1997) found that individuals with more diverse social ties are less susceptible to developing the common cold. There have also been links to acquired immune deficiency syndrome (Klovdahl, 1985), coronary artery disease (Seeman & Syme, 1987), cardiovascular disease (Kawachi et al., 1996), ischemic heart disease, stroke, hypertension, and cancer (Vogt et al., 1992). Helgeson, Cohen, and Fritz (1998) explained the link between social ties and the onset and progression of cancer by suggesting that social ties foster cognitive benefits (e.g., access to information), which is bidirectionally linked to affective benefits such as more positive emotions. Cognitive benefits foster reductions in risk-taking behaviors, screening, timely response to symptoms, and adherence to medicine; and affective behaviors cause a biological response to the neurological and immune system. Together, this pathway affects cancer incidence, survival, mortality, and recurrence (Helgeson et al., 1998). Prospectively, social ties have been linked to breast cancer and colorectal cancer among women. No associations have been found among men or women for lung cancer (Bergelt et al., 2009). However, studies have found either no link between social networks and cancer risk (Eng, Rimm, Fitzmaurice, & Kawachi, 2002; Vogt et al., 1992) or found an association by race (Kinney et al., 2003, 2005) or geography (Iwasaki et al., 2002).

## 4. SOCIAL NETWORKS IN THE DIGITAL AGE: THE LINK TO CANCER

With growing interest in understanding the complex interplay of factors that contribute to health disparities and how to address them, more attention has been placed on the interdependence between people and health. Specifically, studies have explored the health-damaging or health-promoting aspects of social context (Sorensen et al., 2003). In recent years, researchers have began studying the influence of the internet on health because it provides a forum for people to share news, resources, and information, as well as to encourage or discourage health-related behaviors (Evers, 2006). This is largely because behaviors diffuse through social connections and the structure of social networks, thus more studies on the use of social networking (e.g., Myspace, Facebook, Twitter, and Instagram) as an enabler of health have emerged (Centola, 2010; Gold et al., 2011; Greene, Choudhry, Kilabuk, & Shrank, 2011; Kuss & Griffiths, 2011).

People are living longer and technology is advancing. Technological advances have contributed significantly to improvements in cancer. Thus, involving the internet in these efforts is a natural next step. Wantland, Portillo, Holzemer, Slaughter, and McGhee (2004) showed that web-based interventions are effective in behavior change in cancer. Given many cancers are preventable; social media is rapidly becoming an ideal forum to examine knowledge, attitudes, and develop support networks for risk reduction and cancer control (Cavallo, Chou, McQueen, Ramirez, & Riley, 2014). Prior to 2007, social media served as a "sounding board" for both patients and their supporters (Koskan et al., 2014). For example, online cancer support groups have been used as a resource by patients when in-peer support was lacking (Yli-Uotila, Rantanen, & Suominen, 2013); the challenge, however, is the reliability and accuracy of information provided on the internet (e.g., YouTube) (Steinberg et al., 2010).

Although web-based interventions have proven useful for health, the majority of internet users are young adults aged 18–29 and female (74%) (Pew Research Center, 2013). Using online cancer prevention and control interventions among older adults (aged 40+), a group most at-risk of developing cancer, may not be as effective. Older adults use the internet less often than younger adults; thus, they may be less apt to use online social networks over in-person connections. Even with less use of the internet, data show that internet users including older adult users tend to have closer social ties, yet are more socially isolated (Pew Research Center, 2013). For the vast majority of internet users such as adolescents and young adults, online social networking is a viable outlet for understanding health and corresponding behaviors (Yonker, Zan, Scirica, Jethwani, & Kinane, 2015) and enhancing social capital (Pfeil, Arjan, & Zaphiris, 2009). For instance, among non-cancer patients studies report benefits to using social media to relay screening behaviors and information across Twitter (Himelboim & Han, 2014; Lyles, López, Pasick, & Sarkar, 2013; Sugawara et al., 2012). Furthermore, social media is a useful tool for discussing the side effects of medications after diagnosis (Mao et al., 2013). Laranjo et al. (2014) showed that social networking site interventions are effective in changing or improving health behaviors such as physical activity, diet, and smoking cessation. Social media has also been used for the development of cancer control and prevention interventions. QuitNet and the Comprehensive Health Enhancement Support System for Smoking Cessation and Relapse Prevention are two interventions designed to promote smoking cessation (Cobb, Graham, Bock, Papandonatos, & Abrams, 2005; Japuntich et al., 2006) and relapse by providing social support (Japuntich et al., 2006).

As demonstrated, there are a number of web-based programs that have been designed to aid in combating cancer, but accessibility in regards to receiving information and sharing it may not be feasible for all groups as a sole intervention approach. Although the internet is a good source of information for cancer patients (Himelboim & Han, 2014), the Pew Research Center (2013) reports that only 65% of adults 50–64 compared to 89% of teens and young adults use social networking sites. When older adults (60+) do engage socially via the internet, they have less social capital or networks of relationships, compared to teens, yet their pool of friends is more diverse (Pfeil et al., 2009). In addition to dissonance in internet by age, there are also gender differences in the use and benefits of online cancer communities. Although women more than men account for social network users, Durant, McCray, and Safran (2012) found that men prefer to engage socially in large, interconnected, less intimate groups, whereas women desire and prefer more highly intimate bonds and forums that are gender specific. Experience especially with regards to health trumps gender in social engagement. Among cancer survivors, Kim, Wallington, Makambi, and Adams-Campbell (2015) showed that both men and women who talk about health with relatives or friends are more likely to engage in the recommended amount of physical activity. Whether online or in-person, social networks have value in cancer prevention and control and it is the potential of these networks to level the playing field in cancer disparities that warrants research.

## 5. GENDER, CANCER, AND SOCIAL NETWORKS

Gender differences exist in many aspects of life and such differences influence disease and health outcomes. For example, men are more susceptible to developing cancer compared to women (Dorak & Karpuzoglu, 2012). Studies show higher susceptibility among men for 32 out of 35 cancer sites (Edgren, Liang, Adami, & Chang, 2012). For example, age-adjusted cancer mortality rates among men are higher than women, yet 5-year survival rates are lower (Cook, McGlynn, Devesa, Freedman, & Anderson, 2011). A plausible explanation of this disparity is the difference in macrosocial contexts (e.g., social networks) and gendered experiences of males that shape health. Research shows social networks vary by gender (Antonucci, 2001; McLaughlin, Vagenas, Pachana, Begum, & Dobson, 2010; Tucker, Schwartz, Clark, & Friedman, 1999). For instance, women tend to have larger social networks and more network satisfaction than men (McLaughlin et al., 2010). Marital status has been identified as a contributor of this difference, that is, unmarried men (single or divorced) tend to have smaller networks (McLaughlin et al., 2010). Increases in social network size are similar when men and women are widowed (McLaughlin et al., 2010); however, as women age, their social networks are well maintained unlike men.

### 5.1 Networks Among Women

Out of 16 studies, 11 (68.8%) studies were identified in the literature with a focus on social networks among women alone. The most recent studies examined social networks and breast cancer among women postdiagnosis (Beasley et al., 2010; Crookes et al., 2016; Kroenke, Kwan, et al., 2013; Kroenke, Quesenberry, et al., 2013; Kroenke et al., 2012). Earlier studies ($n = 2$) explored the influence of social networks on screening behaviors cross-sectionally (Suarez et al., 1994, 2000). With the exception on one study (Reynolds et al., 1994), participants age range was 40 years or older. Sample sizes ranged from 34 (Crookes et al., 2016) to 4589 (Beasley et al., 2010). Reynolds et al. (1994) found that women with fewer social connections were at greater risk of having later stage disease. Inconsistent findings were observed on the impact of social networks and breast cancer-specific mortality. Beasley et al. (2010) found no association between structural components of networks (e.g., network size and number and frequency of contacts including relatives) and overall or breast cancer-specific survival and mortality, while Kroenke et al. (2012) identified an inverse relationship. Among survivors, socially isolated women had lower scores for physical function than socially integrated women (Michael et al., 2002). Research has also shown that survivors with 0 vs 10 or more close relatives have an increased all-cause and breast cancer mortality and the stage of breast cancer and treatment type were unrelated to social networks (Kroenke et al., 2006). Overall social connectedness is associated with all-cause mortality and frequency of contact with breast cancer-specific mortality (Beasley et al., 2010). This relationship depends on the quality of the relationships that women form with others (Weihs, Enright, & Simmens, 2008). Network members have been identified as a significant predictor of QOL among women with breast cancer (Kroenke, Kwan, et al., 2013); having a larger family network predicts both higher all-cause and breast cancer-specific mortality when participants experience high social burden or high social strain (Kroenke et al., 2012). Studies also show that having more close friends, especially relatives, enhances QOL (Kroenke, Kwan, et al., 2013). Studies examining associations between social networks and QOL among survivors found that socially isolated women were significantly more likely to have lower QOL scores compared to those with less isolation (Kroenke, Kwan, et al., 2013; Michael et al., 2002). Furthermore, prior to diagnosis, isolated women have a twofold increase in breast cancer mortality and 66% all-cause mortality risk (Kroenke et al., 2006). Social networks have also been examined by breast cancer type. The more hours socially isolated women spend in the community and frequent religious services, all-cause mortality decreases (Beasley et al., 2010). Women with invasive breast cancer have a 15–28% reduced risk of death when they are in frequent contact with relatives and friends, attend religious services, and participate in community activities (Beasley et al., 2010). Cancer control literature primarily tackles the importance of downstream factors (e.g., social support) in cancer control. In a systematic review on social support and cancer progression, Nausheen, Gidron, Peveler, and Moss-Morris (2009) found a significant association between social support and progression of breast cancer; however, not among other cancers. Among women survivors, social networks have been specifically linked to health-related QOL and mental health for colorectal cancer (Sapp et al., 2003) and breast cancer (Michael et al., 2002). Social networks have also been linked to cancers that are not gender specific. For example, Lim and Zebrack (2006) observed an indirect association between the size and dependence of social ties and QOL among leukemia and lymphoma patients.

## 5.2 Networks Among Men

In general, men have significantly less healthy lifestyles than women (Antonucci & Akiyama, 1987; Carstensen, 1993). It has been widely recognized that social networks among men and women differ in complex ways, particularly in relation to life stage (Antonucci, 2001; Tucker et al., 1999). Research on social networks among men is limited and the literature on cancer is even rarer. Out of 16 studies included in this review, 1 (6.3%) examined social networks and cancer health specifically among men. Thirty-one percent ($n=5$) included men in the study populations (Bergelt et al., 2009; Chamie et al., 2011; Kinney et al., 2005; Rottenberg et al., 2014; Ye et al., 2009). None of the studies identified in the review reported significant differences in social networks by gender. With the exception of one study (Bergelt et al., 2009), the mean age of men from studies that include men in the sample ranged from 60 to 72. For men, network support is important when making treatment decisions. Men with spouses or in a relationship that have a small network of support (less than two people) were more likely to undergo aggressive treatment (e.g., surgery) than unpartnered men (Chamie et al., 2011). Married men were less likely to have had a colorectal screening test compared to single men (Kinney et al., 2005). Ye et al. (2009) found that a lack of social support from friends and/or relatives influenced men's ability to discuss health and therefore to be screened for colorectal cancer. Domestic studies examining social networks among men are minimal. The majority of studies examining social networks among men have been conducted outside of the United States (Bourne, Morris, Campbell-Smith, & Heaven, 2013; Emerson & Hatton, 2007; Kishi, Eguchi, Sasatani, & Yaguchi, 1994; Rosengren, Orth-Gomer, & Wilhelmsen, 1998; White & Cant, 2003). This may be because other countries recognize the value and relative importance of examining network structures and ties as a "means of reducing inequalities in health" (Acheson et al., 1998). Populations from these studies included both younger and older men. White and Cant (2003) conducted a qualitative assessment of social networks among human immunodeficiency virus (HIV)-positive gay men; study participants reported closer ties through more frequent contact with partners, ex-partners, and friends rather than family members. Bourne et al. (2013) demonstrated that social networks provide men access to health care when no formal health plan is available. Men without health insurance received financial assistance from their social networks to acquire health care. Among men with prostate cancer, Chamie et al. (2011) found that network size (having less than two forms of social support) was associated with undergoing a radical prostatectomy. The probability of choosing surgery was associated with having a partner and no other form of social support. Furthermore, the likelihood of undergoing surgery decreased based upon patients weight, level of education, and D'Amico criteria (PSA level, Gleason score, and clinical stage at diagnosis). The structure of physicians' social networks is also important to cancer disparities among men. Pollack, Weissman, Bekelman, Liao, and Armstrong (2012) found physician social networks influence the access men have to health care providers and treatment options. The similarities of people within these networks thus has the ability to harm or enhance information about risks, prevention, and control of cancer.

## 5.3 Networks and Other Sociodemographic Factors

Gendered experiences or differences in the social experiences of males and females are posited to have a greater effect on social networks (Moen, 2001); however, interpersonal relationships are built upon similarities (McPherson, Smith-Lovin, & Cook, 2001). Socioeconomic factors echo individual and group social experiences produced by social networks; group experiences produce inequalities within personal networks (Campbell, Marsden, & Hurlbert, 1986; McPherson et al., 2001; Moore, 1990) and eventually in health. Seven studies have examined racial and/or socioeconomic differences in social networks (Ajrouch, Antonucci, & Janevic, 2001; Ajrouch, Blandon, & Antonucci, 2005; Chamie et al., 2011; Erwin et al., 2007; Gotay & Wilson, 1998; Kinney et al., 2005; Suarez et al., 1994). Of those studies, two focused on cancer in diverse groups (Kinney et al., 2005; Suarez et al., 1994). In addition to variability in the diversity of social networks among groups (Jones, Cox, & Navarro-Rivera, 2013), the purpose and consistency of social networks vary by race/ethnicity (Cornwell, 2015; Moriarty & Butt, 2004). For instance, research shows that requesting assistance from children when a crisis arises is uncommon among ethnic groups compared to White Americans (Moriarty & Butt, 2004). Strong social networks influence the screening behaviors of racial and ethnic minority women (Gotay & Wilson, 1998; Suarez et al., 1994). Erwin et al. (2007) examined the feasibility of using a tailored intervention model for African American women (Witness Project®) to tailor a breast and cervical cancer education intervention for Latina women. They observed cultural differences and similarities in the primary roles and relationships African Americans play compared to Latina women. Kinney et al. (2005) examined the relationship between structural and functional forms of social ties and colorectal screening by race. Compared to Whites, African Americans were more socially connected and more likely to have undergone a recent colorectal cancer screening (Kinney et al., 2005). Research has shown that African Americans respond to their health based on their social network (Klassen & Washington, 2008). Among African American women, Klassen and Washington (2008) found that social networks influence screening knowledge and religion-based networks are associated with screening behaviors and treatment decisions. African Americans tend to have smaller overall social networks (Jones et al., 2013) and experience more network turnover than Whites (Cornwell, 2015). These findings may be attributed to the high percent of unmarried African Americans compared to Whites (Cantor, Brennan, & Sainz, 1995; Pugliesi & Shook, 1998) or the fact that this group has a shorter life expectancy (Crimmins & Saito, 2001; Ferraro & Farmer, 1996).

## 6. SOCIAL NETWORKS AND HEALTH BEHAVIORS

Social factors foster health behaviors (Christakis & Fowler, 2007; Umberson & Montez, 2010; Ye et al., 2009). Social networks provide a landscape for patients to assemble health information, spread, and develop health behaviors (Christakis & Fowler, 2007; Smith & Christakis, 2008). Granovetter (1973) posits that interactions occurring within networks, particularly small, interpersonal networks provide the "most fruitful" support by shaping, or constraining behavior even when weaker ties exist. Individuals can manipulate their social networks as a means to achieve personal and health goals (Boissevain, 1968; Kapferer, 1969; Mayer, 1966). Christakis (2004) proposed using this dogma to enhance the medical care model by incorporating social ties emphasizing the importance of social contacts and combining sources of information to promote health.

Those with which individuals engage, the choice whether or not to adopt a healthy lifestyle (e.g., not smoking, engaging in routine physical activity) or adhere to recommendations (e.g., fruit and vegetable consumption, cancer screening) or treatments depends on the influence from social networks (Umberson & Montez, 2010). Socially isolated persons are more likely to be smokers, be more sedentary, and have low protein diets (Kroenke et al., 2006). Christakis and Fowler (2007) examined the dynamics of smoking behaviors among offspring from the Framingham Heart Study; they found that friendships decreased the likelihood of smoking by 36%. A personal decision to quit smoking was reflective of group level choices as a result of direct and indirect connections. These outcomes held true up to three degrees of separation (Christakis & Fowler, 2007). Umberson and Montez (2010) equate this influence to the "sense of responsibility" individuals feel for personal and group health, which creates norms that translate into protective health behaviors.

### 6.1 Homophily and Social Networks

Homogeneity within social networks is important to health behaviors. In an assessment of online social networking for breast cancer, Sillence (2013) found that women requested advice on care by targeting "like-minded" people. This type of contact reflects homophily or contact between persons that are similar; the principle of homophily posits that individuals with more similarities engage in frequent contact more often than they do with dissimilar persons and this similarity breeds connections that affect behaviors (McPherson et al., 2001; Pampel, 2002; Phelan, Link, & Tehranifar, 2010). Research shows that social class can impact homophily. For example, a high social class individual can diffuse into the network of a lower class individual causing a change and greater impact than would be anticipated by individuals of their homophilous network alone (DeLamater & Ward, 2013; Rogers, 1995, 2003). Similarities among network members produce inequalities because network members are less likely to engage with members of other networks that may promote the exchange of information and resources necessary to combat adverse health outcomes (Rogers, 1995; Rostila, 2010). Homophily may explain differential burden of disease across groups because health-challenged individuals have less contact with people who can access health information needed to improve, manage, or prevent disease. The information they do receive has little to no influence on behavior (Chang & Lauderdale, 2009; Pampel, Krueger, & Denney, 2010; Phelan et al., 2010).

## 7. DISCUSSION

The relative importance of social networks to cancer disparities hinges on the belief that behaviors and attitudes are shaped by the flow of resources within and opportunities provided by networks. The articles included in this review demonstrate that cancer care behaviors, treatment decisions, and QOL are associated with several aspects of social networks. Resource scarcity coupled with social norms about health, behaviors, and experiences can present a major challenge for socially and economically disadvantaged persons; thus, they are more susceptible to elevated cancer incidence rates and an increased likelihood of late diagnosis (Clegg et al., 2009). Across the social networks and cancer literature, there is consensus that networks are important to overall mortality and important features of these networks (e.g., size, frequency of contact, and member types) enhance or adversely affect health; however, there is a lack of literature examining the role of social networks among groups at higher risk of developing and dying from cancer. Exploring such a social phenomenon may aid in bridging the cancer disparities gap. Furthermore, examining social relationships may provide solution-based public health approaches that could level the playing field in cancer.

## 8. POTENTIAL FOR PUBLIC HEALTH IMPACT

From this review, we know that social connectedness fosters protective health behaviors (e.g., cancer screening) among minorities (Kinney et al., 2005; Suarez et al., 2000; Ye et al., 2009) and QOL among survivors (Kroenke, Kwan, et al., 2013; Michael et al., 2002). In addition, it has an impact on treatment decisions (Chamie et al., 2011) and survival (Reynolds et al., 1994; Rottenberg et al., 2014). When social support is perceived as nonexistent or to be lacking, subjects have worse outcomes such as higher death rates and greater cancer risk compared to those who perceive they have greater social support (Chamie et al., 2011; Reynolds et al., 1994). This review highlights the importance of in-person social networks for cancer prevention and control, given older adults use social media less often and the tools used to measure social networks emphasize in-person interactions. None of the studies in this review examined web-based social networks. Although more than half of the studies in our review included diverse samples, the number of nonwhite subjects was minimal compared to white subjects. Only one study reported differences by race (Chamie et al., 2011). Since minorities, particularly African Americans die disproportionately from many common cancers, oversampling minority groups or designing studies that focus on the social networks of people from these groups may provide more insight into cancer disparities between groups. Without a comparable sample, it is difficult to determine if and what differences exist by sociodemographic factors and doing so is important to address racial and ethnic disparities in cancer. Although the majority (87.5%) of the studies in this review were conducted in the United States, very few were conducted in southern states. The majority of underserved and minority populations reside in the South and cancer rates are also higher in that region. Our findings show the relationship between upstream social factors and health protective (Bergelt et al., 2009) or risk-taking behaviors (Bergelt et al., 2009; Kinney et al., 2005). Understanding the pathways and players that influence outcomes for certain groups have important implications for addressing cancer disparities. This phenomenon is well documented among women for breast cancer, but a major gap exists in the literature among men. More studies on men, particularly on the intentional use of social networks to explore knowledge, attitudes, and beliefs about cancer risk, prevention, and control are needed.

Strong social networks foster important social processes such as education, job opportunities, wealth, and access to healthcare and health behaviors. In addition to health benefits, social networks provide access to invaluable assets including information and resources (Ibarra, 1997) that can either enhance QOL or lead to adverse outcomes. For some groups, social networks include quality resources that foster health advantages, while for others networks produce disadvantage that tends to perpetuate cancer disparities. Medically underserved groups experience disadvantage socially, economically, and environmentally; and this cumulative disadvantage gets under the skin. A substantial literature shows that minorities and low-socioeconomic status (SES) groups meet with challenges when accessing preventive services, including cancer screening which then translates into late stage disease (U.S. Department of Health & Human Services, 2013). Focusing efforts on minorities and low-SES groups and making comparisons with their counterparts will improve our understanding of how social networks can be used to improve access to health care. Sociological and public health researchers must begin to explore how cumulative disadvantage within social networks translates into disparities and how cumulative advantage within networks of the affluent and socially integrated or of nonminority groups can be used to bridge the health disparities gap.

Rothpletz-Puglia, Jones, Storm, Parrott, and O'Brien (2013) examined the feasibility of building social networks for health promotion among women with HIV infection. They found that creating targeted social networks reduces disparities among high risk groups and encourages change in risk-taking behaviors. Personal networks are beneficial when network ties whether formal or informal are strong and resources provided through social networks can be provided when an individual is in need. The impact of these effects vary by the number and type of network members, frequency of engagement and the extent of attachment, geographic proximity, and provision of social support (Ajrouch et al., 2005; Berkman et al., 2000); however, more research in regards to cancer is needed.

Cornwell and Laumann (2013) showed that enhancing personal networks, for example, adding new members can improve functional, self-rated, and psychological health, whereas network losses affect physical health. This may partially explain why African Americans die disproportionately from cancer, yet their White counterparts experience less network turnover (Cornwell, 2015) and have better cancer outcomes. Through social networks, individuals gather and exchange information for themselves as well as others. The silos created by social networks can mean longer, healthier lives for some and lower survival for others.

## 9. CONCLUSIONS

This study provides a brief examination of studies that explored social networks related to cancer. From this review, we know that social networks, an important upstream factor is underexplored in the literature. Social networks whether in-person or online can be used in behavior change interventions; however, tailoring interventions by sociodemographic factors may prove to be more effective. Exploring social networks is an approach that can help to move the needle on health disparities upstream. To further gauge the extent to which social networks influence health behaviors and decision making among adults, a next step would be to explore aspects of networks that may be relevant to the conversation on cancer disparities such as identifying effective methodological approaches used to measure social networks. Future research should also disentangle relationships that exist within social networks and identify ways in which findings can be used to help groups make informed decisions about their health and gain access to appropriate and timely cancer care.

Given adverse health outcomes disproportionately impact individuals with fewer economic resources and less social involvement, characteristics of social networks among these groups have greater implications for developing interventions and strategies that may reduce health disparities and explain marked differences in chronic disease burden. By highlighting the findings in the existing literature, we identified an underdeveloped area of research that could be used to address persistent disparities in cancer. It may especially aid in our understanding of differences between groups, for example, why some groups continue to do progressively well compared to others. This review shows that examining the link between cancer and social networks (structural and functional) is an untapped approach that should be strongly considered to address cancer disparities among vulnerable (e.g., African Americans and other minorities) and understudied populations (e.g., men) nationally and globally.

## REFERENCES

Acheson, D., Barker, D., Chambers, J., Graham, H., Marmot, M., & Whitehead, M. (1998). *Independent inquiry into inequalities in health report.* London: Stationery Office.

Adler, N. E., & Newman, K. (2002). Socioeconomic disparities in health: Pathways and policies. *Health Affairs, 21*(2), 60–76.

Ajrouch, K. J., Antonucci, T. C., & Janevic, M. R. (2001). Social networks among blacks and whites the interaction between race and age. *The Journals of Gerontology. Series B, Psychological Sciences and Social Sciences, 56*(2), S112–S118.

Ajrouch, K. J., Blandon, A. Y., & Antonucci, T. C. (2005). Social networks among men and women: The effects of age and socioeconomic status. *The Journals of Gerontology. Series B, Psychological Sciences and Social Sciences, 60*(6), S311–S317.

Antonucci, T. C. (2001). Social relations: An examination of social networks, social support. *Handbook of the Psychology of Aging, 3*, 427.

Antonucci, T. C., & Akiyama, H. (1987). Social networks in adult life and a preliminary examination of the convoy model. *Journal of Gerontology, 42*(5), 519–527.

Baldwin, L.-M., Dobie, S. A., Billingsley, K., Cai, Y., Wright, G. E., Dominitz, J. A., … Taplin, S. H. (2005). Explaining Black–White differences in receipt of recommended colon cancer treatment. *Journal of the National Cancer Institute, 97*(16), 1211–1220.

Beasley, J. M., Newcomb, P. A., Trentham-Dietz, A., Hampton, J. M., Ceballos, R. M., Titus-Ernstoff, L., … Holmes, M. D. (2010). Social networks and survival after breast cancer diagnosis. *Journal of Cancer Survivorship, 4*(4), 372–380. http://dx.doi.org/10.1007/s11764-010-0139-5.

Bergelt, C., Prescott, E., Gronbaek, M., Koch, U., & Johansen, C. (2009). Social ties and risk for cancer—A prospective cohort study. *Acta Oncologica, 48*(7), 1010–1018. http://dx.doi.org/10.1080/02841860903036230.

Berkman, L. F., & Glass, T. (2000). Social integration, social networks, social support, and health. *Social Epidemiology, 1*, 137–173.

Berkman, L. F., Glass, T., Brissette, I., & Seeman, T. E. (2000). From social integration to health: Durkheim in the new millennium. *Social Science & Medicine, 51*(6), 843–857.

Berkman, L. F., & Syme, S. L. (1979). Social networks, host resistance, and mortality: A nine-year follow-up study of Alameda County residents. *American Journal of Epidemiology, 109*(2), 186–204.

Bhuyan, S. S., Chandak, A., Gupta, N., Isharwal, S., LaGrange, C., Mahmood, A., & Gentry, D. (2015). Patient–provider communication about prostate cancer screening and treatment new evidence from the Health Information National Trends Survey. *American Journal of Men's Health*, 1–13. http://dx.doi.org/10.1177/1557988315614082.

Blazer, D. G. (1982). Social support and mortality in an elderly community population. *American Journal of Epidemiology, 115*(5), 684–694.

Boissevain, J. (1968). The place of non-groups in the social sciences. *Man, 3*(4), 542–556.

Bosworth, H. B., & Schaie, K. W. (1997). The relationship of social environment, social networks, and health outcomes in the Seattle Longitudinal Study: Two analytical approaches. *The Journals of Gerontology Series B, Psychological Sciences and Social Sciences, 52*(5), P197–P205.

Bourne, P. A., Morris, C., Campbell-Smith, J., & Heaven, G. (2013). The role of health status and other variables on social networks among late adult men. *Journal of Behavioral Health, 2*(4), 343–352.

Braveman, P. A., Cubbin, C., Egerter, S., Williams, D. R., & Pamuk, E. (2010). Socioeconomic disparities in health in the United States: What the patterns tell us. *American Journal of Public Health, 100*(S1), S186–S196.

Campbell, K. E., Marsden, P. V., & Hurlbert, J. S. (1986). Social resources and socioeconomic status. *Social Networks, 8*(1), 97–117.

Cantor, M. H., Brennan, M., & Sainz, A. (1995). The importance of ethnicity in the social support systems of older New Yorkers: A longitudinal perspective (1970 to 1990). *Journal of Gerontological Social Work, 22*(3–4), 95–128.

Carstensen, L. L. (1993). Motivation for social contact across the life span: A theory of socioemotional selectivity. In *Paper presented at the Nebraska symposium on motivation.*

Cassel, J. (1976). The contribution of the social environment to host resistance. *American Journal of Epidemiology, 104*(2), 107–123.

Cavallo, D. N., Chou, W.-Y. S., McQueen, A., Ramirez, A., & Riley, W. T. (2014). Cancer prevention and control interventions using social media: User-generated approaches. *Cancer Epidemiology, Biomarkers & Prevention, 23*(9), 1953–1956.

Centola, D. (2010). The spread of behavior in an online social network experiment. *Science, 329*(5996), 1194–1197. http://dx.doi.org/10.1126/science.1185231.

Chamie, K., Kwan, L., Connor, S. E., Zavala, M., Labo, J., & Litwin, M. S. (2011). The impact of social networks and partnership status on treatment choice in men with localized prostate cancer. *BJU International, 109*(7), 1006–1012. http://dx.doi.org/10.1111/j.1464-410X.2011.10515.x.

Chang, V. W., & Lauderdale, D. S. (2009). Fundamental cause theory, technological innovation, and health disparities: The case of cholesterol in the era of statins. *Journal of Health and Social Behavior, 50*(3), 245–260.

Christakis, N. (2004). Social networks and collateral health effects. *BMJ, 329*(7459), 184–185.

Christakis, N. A., & Fowler, J. H. (2007). The spread of obesity in a large social network over 32 years. *New England Journal of Medicine, 357*(4), 370–379.

Clegg, L. X., Reichman, M. E., Miller, B. A., Hankey, B. F., Singh, G. K., Lin, Y. D., … Chen, V. W. (2009). Impact of socioeconomic status on cancer incidence and stage at diagnosis: Selected findings from the surveillance, epidemiology, and end results: National Longitudinal Mortality Study. *Cancer Causes & Control, 20*(4), 417–435.

Cobb, S. (1976). Social support as a moderator of life stress. *Psychosomatic Medicine, 38*(5), 300–314.

Cobb, N. K., Graham, A. L., Bock, B. C., Papandonatos, G., & Abrams, D. B. (2005). Initial evaluation of a real-world Internet smoking cessation system. *Nicotine & Tobacco Research, 7*(2), 207–216.

Cohen, S. (2004). Social relationships and health. *American Psychologist, 59*(8), 676.

Cohen, S., Doyle, W. J., Skoner, D. P., Rabin, B. S., & Gwaltney, J. M. (1997). Social ties and susceptibility to the common cold. *JAMA, 277*(24), 1940–1944.

Cohen, S., & Wills, T. A. (1985). Stress, social support, and the buffering hypothesis. *Psychological Bulletin, 98*(2), 310.

Cook, M. B., McGlynn, K. A., Devesa, S. S., Freedman, N. D., & Anderson, W. F. (2011). Sex disparities in cancer mortality and survival. *Cancer Epidemiology, Biomarkers & Prevention, 20*(8), 1629–1637.

Cornwell, B. (2015). Social disadvantage and network turnover. *The Journals of Gerontology Series B, Psychological Sciences and Social Sciences, 70*(1), 132–142.

Cornwell, B., & Laumann, E. O. (2013). The health benefits of network growth: New evidence from a national survey of older adults. *Social Science & Medicine, 125*, 94–106.

Crimmins, E. M., & Saito, Y. (2001). Trends in healthy life expectancy in the United States, 1970–1990: Gender, racial, and educational differences. *Social Science & Medicine, 52*(11), 1629–1641.

Crookes, D. M., Shelton, R. C., Tehranifar, P., Aycinena, C., Gaffney, A. O., Koch, P., … Greenlee, H. (2016). Social networks and social support for healthy eating among Latina breast cancer survivors: Implications for social and behavioral interventions. *Journal of Cancer Survivorship, 10*(2), 291–301. http://dx.doi.org/10.1007/s11764-015-0475-6.

Davey, S. G., Neaton, J., Wentworth, D., Stamler, R., & Stamler, J. (1998). Mortality differences between black and white men in the USA: Contribution of income and other risk factors among men screened for the MRFIT. MRFIT Research Group. Multiple Risk Factor Intervention Trial. *Lancet, 351*(9107), 934–939.

DeLamater, J. D., & Ward, A. (2013). *Handbook of social psychology*. New York: Springer.

Diderichsen, F., Evans, T., & Whitehead, M. (2001). *The social basis of disparities in health: Challenging inequities in health: From ethics to action*. New York: Oxford University Press.

Dorak, M. T., & Karpuzoglu, E. (2012). Gender differences in cancer susceptibility: An inadequately addressed issue. *Frontiers in Genetics, 3*, 268.

Durant, K. T., McCray, A. T., & Safran, C. (2012). Identifying gender-preferred communication styles within online cancer communities: A retrospective, longitudinal analysis. *PloS One*, 7(11). e49169.

Edgren, G., Liang, L., Adami, H.-O., & Chang, E. T. (2012). Enigmatic sex disparities in cancer incidence. *European Journal of Epidemiology, 27*(3), 187–196.

Emerson, E., & Hatton, C. (2007). Socioeconomic disadvantage, social participation and networks and the self-rated health of English men and women with mild and moderate intellectual disabilities: Cross sectional survey. *European Journal of Public Health, 18*(1), 31–37.

Eng, P. M., Rimm, E. B., Fitzmaurice, G., & Kawachi, I. (2002). Social ties and change in social ties in relation to subsequent total and cause-specific mortality and coronary heart disease incidence in men. *American Journal of Epidemiology, 155*(8), 700–709.

Erwin, D. O., Johnson, V. A., Trevino, M., Duke, K., Feliciano, L., & Jandorf, L. (2007). A comparison of African American and Latina social networks as indicators for culturally tailoring a breast and cervical cancer education intervention. *Cancer, 109*(Suppl. 2), 368–377. http://dx.doi.org/10.1002/cncr.22356.

Evans, S., Metcalfe, C., Ibrahim, F., Persad, R., & Ben-Shlomo, Y. (2008). Investigating Black-White differences in prostate cancer prognosis: A systematic review and meta-analysis. *International Journal of Cancer, 123*(2), 430–435.

Evers, K. E. (2006). eHealth promotion: The use of the Internet for health promotion. *American Journal of Health Promotion, 20*(4), 1–7.

Ferraro, K. F., & Farmer, M. M. (1996). Double jeopardy, aging as leveler, or persistent health inequality? A longitudinal analysis of white and black Americans. *The Journals of Gerontology. Series B, Psychological Sciences and Social Sciences, 51*(6), S319–S328.

Freeman, H. P. (2003). Commentary on the meaning of race in science and society. *Cancer Epidemiology Biomarkers & Prevention, 12*, 232S–236S.

Freeman, H. P., & Chu, K. C. (2005). Determinants of cancer disparities: barriers to cancer screening, diagnosis, and treatment. *Surgical Oncology Clinics of North America, 14*(4), 655–669.

Gerend, M. A., & Pai, M. (2008). Social determinants of black-white disparities in breast cancer mortality: A review. *Cancer Epidemiology, Biomarkers & Prevention, 17*(11), 2913–2923.

Gold, J., Pedrana, A. E., Sacks-Davis, R., Hellard, M. E., Chang, S., Howard, S., … Stoove, M. A. (2011). A systematic examination of the use of online social networking sites for sexual health promotion. *BMC Public Health, 11*(1), 1.

Gotay, C. C., & Wilson, M. (1998). Social support and cancer screening in African American, Hispanic, and Native American women. *Cancer Practice*, *6*(1), 31–37.

Granovetter, M. S. (1973). The strength of weak ties. *American Journal of Sociology*, *78*, 1360–1380.

Greenblatt, M., Becerra, R. M., & Serafetinides, E. (1982). Social networks and mental health: An overview. *The American Journal of Psychiatry*, *139*, 977–984.

Greene, J. A., Choudhry, N. K., Kilabuk, E., & Shrank, W. H. (2011). Online social networking by patients with diabetes: A qualitative evaluation of communication with Facebook. *Journal of General Internal Medicine*, *26*(3), 287–292.

Halbert, C. H., Gattoni-Celli, S., Savage, S., Prasad, S. M., Kittles, R., Briggs, V., ... Johnson, J. C. (2015). Ever and annual use of prostate cancer screening in African American men. *American Journal of Men's Health*. http://dx.doi.org/10.1177/1557988315596225.

Helgeson, V. S., Cohen, S., & Fritz, H. L. (1998). Social ties and cancer. In *Psycho-oncology* (pp. 99–109). Oxford: Oxford University Press.

Himelboim, I., & Han, J. Y. (2014). Cancer talk on twitter: Community structure and information sources in breast and prostate cancer social networks. *Journal of Health Communication*, *19*(2), 210–225. http://dx.doi.org/10.1080/10810730.2013.811321.

Holt-Lunstad, J., Smith, T. B., & Layton, J. B. (2010). Social relationships and mortality risk: A meta-analytic review. *PLoS Medicine*, 7(7). e1000316.

House, J. S., Landis, K. R., & Umberson, D. (1988). Social relationships and health. *Science*, *241*(4865), 540–545.

Ibarra, H. (1997). Paving an alternative route: Gender differences in managerial networks. *Social Psychology Quarterly*, *60*, 91–102.

Institute of Medicine (2003). Unequal treatment: Confronting racial and ethnic disparities in healthcare. Washington, DC: The National Academies Press.

Iwasaki, M., Otani, T., Sunaga, R., Miyazaki, H., Xiao, L., Wang, N., ... Suzuki, S. (2002). Social networks and mortality based on the Komo-Ise cohort study in Japan. *International Journal of Epidemiology*, *31*(6), 1208–1218.

Japuntich, S. J., Zehner, M. E., Smith, S. S., Jorenby, D. E., Valdez, J. A., Fiore, M. C., ... Gustafson, D. H. (2006). Smoking cessation via the internet: A randomized clinical trial of an internet intervention as adjuvant treatment in a smoking cessation intervention. *Nicotine & Tobacco Research*, *8*(Suppl. 1), S59–S67.

Jepson, C., Kessler, L. G., Portnoy, B., & Gibbs, T. (1991). Black-white differences in cancer prevention knowledge and behavior. *American Journal of Public Health*, *81*(4), 501–504.

Jones, R. P., Cox, D., & Navarro-Rivera, J. (2013). *The 2013 American values survey: In search of libertarians in America*. Washington, DC: Religion Research Institute.

Kapferer, B. (1969). *Norms and the manipulation of relationships in a work context*. Manchester: Manchester University Press.

Kawachi, I., & Berkman, L. F. (2001). Social ties and mental health. *Journal of Urban Health*, *78*(3), 458–467.

Kawachi, I., Colditz, G. A., Ascherio, A., Rimm, E. B., Giovannucci, E., Stampfer, M. J., & Willett, W. C. (1996). A prospective study of social networks in relation to total mortality and cardiovascular disease in men in the USA. *Journal of Epidemiology and Community Health*, *50*(3), 245–251.

Kim, B. H., Wallington, S. F., Makambi, K. H., & Adams-Campbell, L. L. (2015). Social networks and physical activity behaviors among cancer survivors: Data from the 2005 Health Information National Trends Survey. *Journal of Health Communication*, *20*(6), 656–662. http://dx.doi.org/10.1080/10810730.2015.1018576.

Kinlock, B. L., Thorpe, R. J., Jr., Howard, D. L., Bowie, J. V., Ross, L. E., Fakunle, D. O., & LaVeist, T. A. (2016). Racial disparity in time between first diagnosis and initial treatment of prostate cancer. *Cancer Control: Journal of the Moffitt Cancer Center*, *23*(1), 47–51.

Kinney, A. Y., Bloor, L. E., Dudley, W. N., Millikan, R. C., Marshall, E., Martin, C., & Sandler, R. S. (2003). Roles of religious involvement and social support in the risk of colon cancer among blacks and whites. *American Journal of Epidemiology, 158*(11), 1097–1107.

Kinney, A. Y., Bloor, L. E., Martin, C., & Sandler, R. S. (2005). Social ties and colorectal cancer screening among Blacks and Whites in North Carolina. *Cancer Epidemiology, Biomarkers and Prevention, 14*(1), 182–189.

Kishi, R., Eguchi, T., Sasatani, H., & Yaguchi, T. (1994). Health status, social networks and support systems of elderly men and women in a large city and in former coal-mining areas—A population-based comparative study of 70-year-old residents of Sapporo and Yubari. *[Nihon koshu eisei zasshi] Japanese Journal of Public Health, 41*(5), 474–488.

Klassen, A. C., & Washington, C. (2008). How does social integration influence breast cancer control among urban African-American women? Results from a cross-sectional survey. *BMC Women's Health, 8*(4), 1–10.

Klovdahl, A. S. (1985). Social networks and the spread of infectious diseases: The AIDS example. *Social Science & Medicine, 21*(11), 1203–1216.

Klovdahl, A. S., Potterat, J. J., Woodhouse, D. E., Muth, J. B., Muth, S. Q., & Darrow, W. W. (1994). Social networks and infectious disease: The Colorado Springs study. *Social Science & Medicine, 38*(1), 79–88.

Kohler, B. A., Sherman, R. L., Howlader, N., Jemal, A., Ryerson, A. B., Henry, K. A., … Noone, A.-M. (2015). Annual report to the nation on the status of cancer, 1975–2011, featuring incidence of breast cancer subtypes by race/ethnicity, poverty, and state. *Journal of the National Cancer Institute, 107*(6), djv048.

Koskan, A., Klasko, L., Davis, S. N., Gwede, C. K., Wells, K. J., Kumar, A., … Meade, C. D. (2014). Use and taxonomy of social media in cancer-related research: A systematic review. *American Journal of Public Health, 104*(7), e20–e37.

Kroenke, C. H., Kubzansky, L. D., Schernhammer, E. S., Holmes, M. D., & Kawachi, I. (2006). Social networks, social support, and survival after breast cancer diagnosis. *Journal of Clinical Oncology, 24*(7), 1105–1111. http://dx.doi.org/10.1200/jco.2005.04.2846.

Kroenke, C. H., Kwan, M. L., Neugut, A. I., Ergas, I. J., Wright, J. D., Caan, B. J., … Kushi, L. H. (2013). Social networks, social support mechanisms, and quality of life after breast cancer diagnosis. *Breast Cancer Research and Treatment, 139*(2), 515–527. http://dx.doi.org/10.1007/s10549-013-2477-2.

Kroenke, C. H., Michael, Y., Tindle, H., Gage, E., Chlebowski, R., Garcia, L., … Caan, B. J. (2012). Social networks, social support and burden in relationships, and mortality after breast cancer diagnosis. *Breast Cancer Research and Treatment, 133*(1), 375–385. http://dx.doi.org/10.1007/s10549-012-1962-3.

Kroenke, C. H., Quesenberry, C., Kwan, M. L., Sweeney, C., Castillo, A., & Caan, B. J. (2013). Social networks, social support, and burden in relationships, and mortality after breast cancer diagnosis in the Life After Breast Cancer Epidemiology (LACE) study. *Breast Cancer Research and Treatment, 137*(1), 261–271. http://dx.doi.org/10.1007/s10549-012-2253-8.

Kuss, D. J., & Griffiths, M. D. (2011). Online social networking and addiction—A review of the psychological literature. *International Journal of Environmental Research and Public Health, 8*(9), 3528–3552.

Laranjo, L., Arguel, A., Neves, A. L., Gallagher, A. M., Kaplan, R., Mortimer, N., … Lau, A. Y. (2014). The influence of social networking sites on health behavior change: A systematic review and meta-analysis. *Journal of the American Medical Informatics Association, 22*(1), 243–256.

Li, C. I., Malone, K. E., & Daling, J. R. (2003). Differences in breast cancer stage, treatment, and survival by race and ethnicity. *Archives of Internal Medicine, 163*(1), 49–56.

Lim, J. W., & Zebrack, B. (2006). Social networks and quality of life for long-term survivors of leukemia and lymphoma. *Support Care Cancer, 14*(2), 185–192. http://dx.doi.org/10.1007/s00520-005-0856-x.
Lyles, C. R., López, A., Pasick, R., & Sarkar, U. (2013). 5 mins of uncomfyness is better than dealing with cancer 4 a lifetime: An exploratory qualitative analysis of cervical and breast cancer screening dialogue on Twitter. *Journal of Cancer Education, 28*(1), 127–133.
Mao, J. J., Chung, A., Benton, A., Hill, S., Ungar, L., Leonard, C. E., ... Holmes, J. H. (2013). Online discussion of drug side effects and discontinuation among breast cancer survivors. *Pharmacoepidemiology and Drug Safety, 22*(3), 256–262.
Mayer, A. (1966). The significance of quasi-groups in the study of complex societies. In M. Banton (Ed.), *The social anthropology of complex societies* (pp. 97–122). Abingdon, Oxon: Routledge.
McLaughlin, D., Vagenas, D., Pachana, N. A., Begum, N., & Dobson, A. (2010). Gender differences in social network size and satisfaction in adults in their 70s. *Journal of Health Psychology, 15*(5), 671–679.
McPherson, M., Smith-Lovin, L., & Cook, J. M. (2001). Birds of a feather: Homophily in social networks. *Annual Review of Sociology, 27*, 415–444.
Mead, H., Cartwright-Smith, L., Jones, K., Ramos, C., Woods, K., & Siegel, B. (2008). *Racial and ethnic disparities in US health care: A chartbook*. New York, NY: The Commonwealth Fund.
Michael, Y. L., Berkman, L. F., Colditz, G. A., Holmes, M. D., & Kawachi, I. (2002). Social networks and health-related quality of life in breast cancer survivors: A prospective study. *Journal of Psychosomatic Research, 52*(5), 285–293.
Moen, P. (2001). The gendered life course. In R. H. G. Binstock & K. Linda (Eds.), *Handbook of aging and the social sciences*. (5th ed.). San Diego, CA: Academic Press.
Moore, G. (1990). Structural determinants of men's and women's personal networks. *American Sociological Review, 55*, 726–735.
Moriarty, J., & Butt, J. (2004). Inequalities in quality of life among older people from different ethnic groups. *Ageing and Society, 24*(05), 729–753.
Nausheen, B., Gidron, Y., Peveler, R., & Moss-Morris, R. (2009). Social support and cancer progression: A systematic review. *Journal of Psychosomatic Research, 67*(5), 403–415.
Orth-Gomer, K., & Johnson, J. V. (1987). Social network interaction and mortality: A six year follow-up study of a random sample of the Swedish population. *Journal of Chronic Diseases, 40*(10), 949–957.
Pampel, F. C. (2002). Inequality, diffusion, and the status gradient in smoking. *Social Problems, 49*(1), 35–57.
Pampel, F. C., Krueger, P. M., & Denney, J. T. (2010). Socioeconomic disparities in health behaviors. *Annual Review of Sociology, 36*, 349.
Pew Research Center. (2013). *Social networking fact sheet*. Washington, DC: PR Center.
Pfeil, U., Arjan, R., & Zaphiris, P. (2009). Age differences in online social networking—A study of user profiles and the social capital divide among teenagers and older users in MySpace. *Computers in Human Behavior, 25*(3), 643–654.
Phelan, J. C., Link, B. G., & Tehranifar, P. (2010). Social conditions as fundamental causes of health inequalities theory, evidence, and policy implications. *Journal of Health and Social Behavior, 51*(Suppl. 1), S28–S40.
Pinquart, M., & Duberstein, P. R. (2010). Associations of social networks with cancer mortality: A meta-analysis. *Critical Reviews in Oncology/Hematology, 75*(2), 122–137. http://dx.doi.org/10.1016/j.critrevonc.2009.06.003.
Pollack, C. E., Weissman, G., Bekelman, J., Liao, K., & Armstrong, K. (2012). Physician social networks and variation in prostate cancer treatment in three cities. *Health Services Research, 47*(1 Pt. 2), 380–403. http://dx.doi.org/10.1111/j.1475-6773.2011.01331.x.

Pugliesi, K., & Shook, S. L. (1998). Gender, ethnicity, and network characteristics: Variation in social support resources 1. *Sex Roles*, *38*(3–4), 215–238.

Reynolds, P., Boyd, P. T., Blacklow, R. S., Jackson, J. S., Greenberg, R. S., Austin, D. F., ... Edwards, B. K. (1994). The relationship between social ties and survival among black and white breast cancer patients. National Cancer Institute Black/White Cancer Survival Study Group. *Cancer Epidemiology, Biomarkers and Prevention*, *3*(3), 253–259.

Reynolds, P., & Kaplan, G. A. (1990). Social connections and risk for cancer: Prospective evidence from the Alameda County Study. *Behavioral Medicine*, *16*(3), 101–110.

Rogers, E. M. (1995). *Diffusion of innovations* (4th ed.). New York: Simon and Schuster.

Rogers, E. M. (2003). *Diffusion of innovations* (5th ed.). New York: Simon and Schuster.

Rosengren, A., Orth-Gomer, K., & Wilhelmsen, L. (1998). Socioeconomic differences in health indices, social networks and mortality among Swedish men. A study of men born in 1933. *Scandinavian Journal of Public Health*, *26*(4), 272–280.

Rostila, M. (2010). Birds of a feather flock together—And fall ill? Migrant homophily and health in Sweden. *Sociology of Health & Illness*, *32*(3), 382–399.

Rothpletz-Puglia, P., Jones, V. M., Storm, D. S., Parrott, J. S., & O'Brien, K. A. (2013). Peer reviewed: Building social networks for health promotion: Shout-out health, New Jersey, 2011. *Preventing Chronic Disease*, *10*, E147.

Rottenberg, Y., Litwin, H., Manor, O., Paltiel, A., Barchana, M., & Paltiel, O. (2014). Prediagnostic self-assessed health and extent of social networks predict survival in older individuals with cancer: A population based cohort study. *Journal of Geriatric Oncology*, *5*(4), 400–407.

Ryerson A. B., Eheman C. R., Altekruse S. F., Ward J. W., Jemal, A., Sherman, R. L., ... Kohler, B. A. (2016). Annual report to the Nation on the Status of Cancer, 1975–2012, featuring the increasing incidence of liver cancer, 2016, *Public Health Resources*, Paper 468.

Sapp, A. L., Trentham-Dietz, A., Newcomb, P. A., Hampton, J. M., Moinpour, C. M., & Remington, P. L. (2003). Social networks and quality of life among female long-term colorectal cancer survivors. *Cancer*, *98*(8), 1749–1758.

Seeman, T. E. (1996). Social ties and health: The benefits of social integration. *Annals of Epidemiology*, *6*(5), 442–451.

Seeman, T. E., & Syme, S. L. (1987). Social networks and coronary artery disease: A comparison of the structure and function of social relations as predictors of disease. *Psychosomatic Medicine*, *49*(4), 341–354.

Shavers, V. L., & Brown, M. L. (2002). Racial and ethnic disparities in the receipt of cancer treatment. *Journal of the National Cancer Institute*, *94*(5), 334–357.

Shavers, V. L., Brown, M. L., Potosky, A. L., Klabunde, C. N., Davis, W., Moul, J. W., & Fahey, A. (2004). Race/ethnicity and the receipt of watchful waiting for the initial management of prostate cancer. *Journal of General Internal Medicine*, *19*(2), 146–155.

Siegel, R. L., Miller, K. D., & Jemal, A. (2016). Cancer statistics, 2016. *CA: A Cancer Journal for Clinicians*, *66*(1), 7–30.

Sillence, E. (2013). Giving and receiving peer advice in an online breast cancer support group. *Cyberpsychology, Behavior, and Social Networking*, *16*(6), 480–485.

Smith, K. P., & Christakis, N. A. (2008). Social networks and health. *Annual Review of Sociology*, *34*, 405–429.

Smith, E. C., Ziogas, A., & Anton-Culver, H. (2013). Delay in surgical treatment and survival after breast cancer diagnosis in young women by race/ethnicity. *JAMA Surgery*, *148*(6), 516–523.

Song, L., Weaver, M. A., Chen, R. C., Bensen, J. T., Fontham, E., Mohler, J. L., ... Sleath, B. (2014). Associations between patient–provider communication and socio-cultural factors in prostate cancer patients: A cross-sectional evaluation of racial differences. *Patient Education and Counseling*, *97*(3), 339–346.

Sorensen, G., Emmons, K., Hunt, M. K., Barbeau, E., Goldman, R., Peterson, K., … Berkman, L. (2003). Model for incorporating social context in health behavior interventions: Applications for cancer prevention for working-class, multiethnic populations. *Preventive Medicine*, *37*(3), 188–197.
Steinberg, P. L., Wason, S., Stern, J. M., Deters, L., Kowal, B., & Seigne, J. (2010). YouTube as source of prostate cancer information. *Urology*, *75*(3), 619–622.
Stokes, W. A., Hendrix, L. H., Royce, T. J., Allen, I. M., Godley, P. A., & Wang, A. Z. (2013). Racial differences in time from prostate cancer diagnosis to treatment initiation. *Cancer*, *119*(13), 2486–2493.
Suarez, L., Lloyd, L., Weiss, N., Rainbolt, T., & Pulley, L. (1994). Effect of social networks on cancer-screening behavior of older Mexican-American women. *Journal of the National Cancer Institute*, *86*(10), 775–779.
Suarez, L., Ramirez, A. G., Villarreal, R., Marti, J., McAlister, A., Talavera, G. A., … Perez-Stable, E. J. (2000). Social networks and cancer screening in four US Hispanic groups. *American Journal of Preventive Medicine*, *19*(1), 47–52.
Sugawara, Y., Narimatsu, H., Hozawa, A., Shao, L., Otani, K., & Fukao, A. (2012). Cancer patients on Twitter: A novel patient community on social media. *BMC Research Notes*, *5*(1), 699.
Thoits, P. A. (2011). Mechanisms linking social ties and support to physical and mental health. *Journal of Health and Social Behavior*, *52*(2), 145–161.
Thomas, B. C., Groff, S. L., Tsang, K., & Carlson, L. E. (2009). Patient ethnicity: A key predictor of cancer care satisfaction. *Ethnicity & Health*, *14*(4), 351–358.
Tucker, J. S., Schwartz, J. E., Clark, K. M., & Friedman, H. S. (1999). Age-related changes in the associations of social network ties with mortality risk. *Psychology and Aging*, *14*(4), 564.
U.S. Department of Health & Human Services (2011). *Healthy people 2020*. Washington, DC: US Department of Health and Human Services. 2010.
U.S. Department of Health & Human Services (2013). *2012 National healthcare disparities report*. Rockville, MD: Agency for Healthcare Research and Quality.
Umberson, D., & Montez, J. K. (2010). Social relationships and health a flashpoint for health policy. *Journal of Health and Social Behavior*, *51*(Suppl. 1), S54–S66.
Vogt, T. M., Mullooly, J. P., Ernst, D., Pope, C. R., & Hollis, J. F. (1992). Social networks as predictors of ischemic heart disease, cancer, stroke and hypertension: Incidence, survival and mortality. *Journal of Clinical Epidemiology*, *45*(6), 659–666.
Wantland, D. J., Portillo, C. J., Holzemer, W. L., Slaughter, R., & McGhee, E. M. (2004). The effectiveness of web-based vs. non-web-based interventions: A meta-analysis of behavioral change outcomes. *Journal of Medical Internet Research*, *6*(4). e40.
Weihs, K. L., Enright, T. M., & Simmens, S. J. (2008). Close relationships and emotional processing predict decreased mortality in women with breast cancer: Preliminary evidence. *Psychosomatic Medicine*, *70*(1), 117–124.
White, L., & Cant, B. (2003). Social networks, social support, health and HIV-positive gay men. *Health & Social Care in the Community*, *11*(4), 329–334.
Williams, D. R., & Jackson, P. B. (2005). Social sources of racial disparities in health. *Health Affairs*, *24*(2), 325–334.
Wolf, A., Wender, R. C., Etzioni, R. B., Thompson, I. M., D'Amico, A. V., Volk, R. J., … Andrews, K. (2010). American Cancer Society guideline for the early detection of prostate cancer: Update 2010. *CA: A Cancer Journal for Clinicians*, *60*(2), 70–98.
Woolf, S. H., & Braveman, P. (2011). Where health disparities begin: The role of social and economic determinants—And why current policies may make matters worse. *Health Affairs*, *30*(10), 1852–1859.
Ye, J., Williams, S. D., & Xu, Z. (2009). The association between social networks and colorectal cancer screening in American males and females: Data from the 2005 Health

Information National Trends Survey. *Cancer Causes and Control, 20*(7), 1227–1233. http://dx.doi.org/10.1007/s10552-009-9335-x.

Yli-Uotila, T., Rantanen, A., & Suominen, T. (2013). Motives of cancer patients for using the Internet to seek social support. *European Journal of Cancer Care, 22*(2), 261–271.

Yonker, L. M., Zan, S., Scirica, C. V., Jethwani, K., & Kinane, T. B. (2015). "Friending" teens: Systematic review of social media in adolescent and young adult health care. *Journal of Medical Internet Research, 17*(1), e4.

CHAPTER SIX

# Disparities in Cervical Cancer Incidence and Mortality: Can Epigenetics Contribute to Eliminating Disparities?

**R.L. Maguire*, A.C. Vidal†, S.K. Murphy‡, C. Hoyo*,[1]**
*North Carolina State University, Raleigh, NC, United States
†Cedar-Sinai Medical Center, Los Angeles, CA, United States
‡Duke University Medical Center, Durham, NC, United States
[1]Corresponding author: e-mail address: choyo@ncsu.edu

## Contents



## Abstract

Screening for uterine cervical intraepithelial neoplasia (CIN) followed by aggressive treatment has reduced invasive cervical cancer (ICC) incidence and mortality. However, ICC cases and carcinoma in situ (CIS) continue to be diagnosed annually in the United States, with minorities bearing the brunt of this burden. Because ICC peak incidence and

*Advances in Cancer Research*, Volume 133
ISSN 0065-230X
http://dx.doi.org/10.1016/bs.acr.2016.09.001

mortality are 10–15 years earlier than other solid cancers, the number of potential years of life lost to this cancer is substantial. Screening for early signs of CIN is still the mainstay of many cervical cancer control programs. However, the accuracy of existing screening tests remains suboptimal. Changes in epigenetic patterns that occur as a result of human papillomavirus infection contribute to CIN progression to cancer, and can be harnessed to improve existing screening tests. However, this requires a concerted effort to identify the epigenomic landscape that is reliably altered by HPV infection specific to ICC, distinct from transient changes.

## 1. INTRODUCTION

Screening for uterine cervical intraepithelial neoplasia (CIN) and treating these aggressively has reduced invasive cervical cancer (ICC) incidence and mortality. However, nearly 13,000 ICC cases and >40,000 cases of carcinoma in situ (CIS) continue to be diagnosed annually in the United States alone (Jemal et al., 2011). Because ICC peak incidence and mortality are 10–15 years earlier than other cancers, the number of potential years of life lost to this cancer is substantial (Franco, Schlecht, & Saslow, 2003; Goldstein, Bray, Parkin, Sellors, & Zhang, 2010). While an estimated 55% of incident ICC is due to insufficient screening, a proportion almost as large is due to detection failure (~30%), and incomplete follow-up (~13%) after lesions are identified (Schiffman & Solomon, 2003). This suboptimal accuracy of existing testing and triage guidelines generates >2 million cases with abnormal cytological findings that must be followed for periods of up to 2 years, at great cost to the individual and the healthcare system (Schiffman & Adrianza, 2000). This inaccuracy is also hypothesized to contribute to poor adherence to recommended follow-up care, more frequently reported in poor-resourced settings (Eggleston, Coker, Luchok, & Meyer, 2007; Schiffman & Adrianza, 2000; Wordlaw-Stinson et al., 2014).

Stable DNA methylation changes in *cis*-acting differentially methylated regions (DMRs) that regulate imprinted gene expression have been implicated in cancer initiation and progression (Jirtle, 1999, 2009; Jirtle & Skinner, 2007). The purpose of this review is to summarize available data on disparities of cervical cancer and host DNA methylation patterns. We then assess the extent to which these patterns can be used to improve screening algorithms to decrease the incidence and mortality of cervical cancer.

## 2. DISPARITIES IN CERVICAL CANCER INCIDENCE AND MORTALITY

Screening for early signs of uterine CIN and aggressive treatment has led to major reductions in ICC incidence and mortality. However, globally, approximately half a million cases continue to be diagnosed and >270,000 deaths continue to occur each year, making ICC the third most common cause of cancer-related death among women, and the top cancer killer among women in developing countries (Goldstein et al., 2010). In the United States of the nearly 13,000 ICC cases, >40,000 cases of CIS, and 4100 deaths that are reported annually, ethnic minorities and women of lower socioeconomic status (SES) are at higher risk (American Cancer Society, 2005).

The incidence among African Americans is >60% higher compared to European American women, and the risk of later stage at diagnosis and death is more than double that of European Americans (American Cancer Society, 2005, 2012; Porterfield, Dutton, & Gizlice, 2003; Smith, 2008; Smith et al., 2003, 2007). Moreover, cervical cancer-related mortality is higher in African Americans than Hispanics or European Americans (Smith, 2008). These disparities are despite high acceptability of the screening test (i.e., the coverage exceeds 80% of the eligible US population), comparable screening rates to detect precancerous lesions and similar prevalence of human papillomavirus (HPV) infection overall. These disparities are also despite lower prevalence of cofactors for ICC among minorities, such as cigarette smoking and oral contraceptive use in women aged <25 years. While HPV vaccination rates have been increasing in the United States, coverage remains low: ~40% of female children 13–17 years have received the three doses of the vaccine (Markowitz et al., 2016; Torre, Siegel, Ward, & Jemal, 2016).

The picture globally is similar with more than 80% of cervical cancer deaths being reported in low- and middle-income countries, where vaccine costs remain prohibitive. In fact, the World Health Organization estimates that the incidence of cervical cancer will be 40% higher by 2030, with most of the cases diagnosed in low- and middle-income countries (Torre et al., 2016). Because ICC peak incidence and mortality are between ages 45 and 60 years, i.e., 10–15 years earlier than other solid cancers, this cancer ranks as the fourth highest in the number of potential years of life lost in the United States (Franco et al., 2003; Goldstein et al., 2010).

## 3. DISPARITIES IN CIN INCIDENCE

Although there are no population-based registries from which incidence data on the full spectrum of precursor lesions can be discerned nationally, up until 5 years ago, the general consensus was that in the United States, the incidence of precursor lesions was on the increase, an increase that some suggest is due to a cohort effect or rise in the incidence of adenocarcinomas (Chan, Sung, & Sawaya, 2003; Franco, 2003; Franco, Duarte-Franco, & Ferenczy, 2001); the increase was also steeper in African Americans (Franco & Ferenczy, 2002; Sigurdsson, 1999). However, recent data from surveillance areas of two east coast and two west coast states of the United States suggest that the incidence which ranged by age from 293/100,000 to 407/1000 was highest in European Americans and lowest in Asian Americans. While this incidence was generally on the decline between 2008 and 2012, this change is largely driven by the declining incidence among younger women where vaccine uptake is also highest; it remains unchanged in women aged 30–39 years (Hariri et al., 2015). However, the majority of women diagnosed with intraepithelial neoplasia do not progress to invasive cancer. Factors associated with progression from CIN to cancer include infection with HPV—the etiologic agent for this cancer, together with cofactors. The established cofactors are cigarette smoking, higher parity, long duration of hormonal contraceptive use, and poor adherence to recommended screening.

## 4. HUMAN PAPILLOMAVIRUS

It is generally agreed that infection with sexually transmitted human papillomavirus (HPV) is a necessary but not sufficient cause of CIN2+ (Becker et al., 1991; Bosch et al., 1993; Coker et al., 1993; Kadish et al., 1992; Koutsky et al., 1992; Levine et al., 1993; Morrison et al., 1991; Schiff et al., 2000; van den Brule et al., 1992; Wallboomers et al., 1999). Of the more than 200 HPV genotypes, less than 40 harbor in the genital tract, and are categorized as *high-risk*, *intermediate-risk*, or *low-risk* HPV genotypes, depending on the magnitude of their association with squamous cell carcinoma of the uterine cervix.

Mechanisms by which HPV infection causes cancer have been known for some time, and are well described. Following infection with *low-risk* HPV subtypes including 6, 11, 42, 43, and 44, the viral DNA persists in circular form and is maintained as episomal DNA (Arends, Buckley, & Wells, 1998). Factors associated with HPV DNA integration into the host genome are largely unknown, although immune competence (Hernandez, McDuffie, Franke, Killeen, & Goodman, 2004; Schiffman et al., 1993) and older age are thought to contribute significantly. However, following infection with subtypes classified as *high-risk* (HPV16 and 18) or *intermediate risk* (HPV31, 33, 35, 39, 45, 51, 52, 56, 58, 59, and 68), the viral DNA persists in circular form only until the disruption of its E2 region, which allows integration of its DNA into the host genome (Arends et al., 1998). Such integration is thought to occur at methylation-sensitive sites (Hernandez et al., 2004). Indeed, genomes of *high-risk* HPVs are found integrated into the cellular DNA in most CIN2+ cases, including in situ and invasive cancer (Choo et al., 1987; Schiffman et al., 1993).

Younger age is consistent risk factors for HPV infection. A National Health and Nutrition Examination Survey (NHANES) analysis (Dunne et al., 2007) suggested that the prevalence of HPV infection is inversely related to age, with the highest rates among women aged 20–24 years and the lowest among women aged 50–59 years. This difference in HPV prevalence by age has remained unchanged, although it is much lower in women younger than 20 years presumably owing to the vaccine (Markowitz et al., 2016). Although the prevalence of *any HPV* infection is higher in African Americans (39%), there seems to be no sizable ethnic/race differences in the prevalence of *high-risk* or *intermediate-risk* HPV subtypes (Kahn, Lan, & Kahn, 2007). However, the majority of women infected with *high-risk* HPV do not develop CIN, and even fewer develop cancer. Thus, screening for intraepithelial lesions is the mainstay of cervical cancer control programs globally.

## 5. SCREENING

Although screening and aggressive treatment has reduced cancer incidence, clinically utilized screening tests based on cytopathology augmented with detection of high-risk (HR)-HPV (Schiffman & Adrianza, 2000) generate a large number of false negatives and false positives requiring protracted follow-up care. To improve the accuracy of current screening strategies, a risk score-based system (Hoyo, Miller, Newman, & Fortney, 2000), visual inspection of the aceto-white cervix (Chumworathayi, Eamratsameekool, Kularbkaew, & Chumworathayi, 2008; University of Zimbabwe/JHPIEGO Cervical Cancer Project, 1999), and other visual aids currently in clinical trials have been proposed. Also, several studies (Cortecchia et al., 2013; del Pino et al., 2009; Hariri & Oster, 2007; Liao et al., 2014; Mills, Paquette, Castle, & Stoler, 2015; Ozaki, Zen, & Inoue, 2011; Pacchiarotti et al., 2014; Sagasta et al., 2016) have evaluated the utility of p16 staining (currently used to identify CIN2+) in identifying CIN1 likely to progress. Results are conflicting and show wide range in sensitivity (50–100%), specificity (37–72%), and positive predictive value of 10–35% (Cortecchia et al., 2013; del Pino et al., 2009; Hariri & Oster, 2007; Liao et al., 2014; Mills et al., 2015; Ozaki et al., 2011; Pacchiarotti et al., 2014; Sagasta et al., 2016). This has led some (Sagasta et al., 2016) to conclude that p16 has limited value in discriminating CIN1 likely to progress.

Collectively, these efforts attest to a need to develop new ways to better discriminate lesions likely to progress to invasive cancer. While the new HPV vaccine will eventually decrease the prevalence of ICC in the future, it is unlikely to reduce incidence in women aged >25 years, as the vaccination rates decrease with increasing age (Hariri et al., 2015) even after extensive education (Ferris, Waller, Owen, & Smith, 2007); this proportion is even lower in women of lower SES, who also are at higher invasive cancer risk.

## 6. COFACTORS OF HPV INFECTION AND CIN PROGRESSION

In addition to HPV subtype and older age at infection, cofactors associated with progression have been an active topic of research for some time, and include: adherence to follow-up evaluation and treatment recommendations following screening, cigarette smoking, long-term oral contraceptive use, high parity, and nutritional deficiency where folate levels are the most intensively investigated. Below, we summarize evidence for associations between putative cofactors associated with progression to CIN2 or worse among women infected with "high" or "intermediate" HPV subtypes that may explain the preponderance of poorer outcomes among African Americans. We then posit the hypothesis of multigenerational effects of cofactors and deregulation of regulatory elements of epigenetically labile regulatory regions and risk of cancer or progression to CIN2 or worse.

### 6.1 Poor Adherence to Recommended Care in Ethnic Minorities

Poor adherence to screening to detect precursor lesions early, and to follow-up recommendations following abnormal screening tests has been hypothesized as key in explaining poorer outcomes among African Americans with comparable "high-risk" or "intermediate-risk" HPV infection rates (Eggleston et al., 2007). However, recent data do not support that the incidence in CIN2+ can be explained health-care access, defined by having insurance (Hariri et al., 2015). In the United States, another study found similar survival rates in African American and European American women of similar ages and stage at diagnoses, enrolled in the military health-care system where access to follow-up care is independent of ability to pay (Farley et al., 2001).

The link between poor adherence to recommendations and lower SES has led to the conclusion that limited ability to pay for follow-up treatment underlies progression to CIN2+ (Eggleston et al., 2007; Franco et al., 2001). That African Americans are less likely to receive intensive therapy (Akers, Newmann, & Smith, 2007) due to advanced disease at diagnosis has also been hypothesized as a potential explanation for higher mortality among this group. This notion is supported by findings that African American women are two times more likely than European American women to receive a diagnosis of distant ICC (Saraiya et al., 2007), although this could also be due to a more aggressive course of tumorigenesis. However, Hispanics, who also have poor access to follow-up care, and have comparable "high" and "intermediate" risk HPV infection rates, have lower CIS and ICC incidence and ICC-related mortality. Furthermore, screening rates to identify precursor lesions are overall higher in African American than in Hispanic or in European American women (although slightly lower in women aged 45 years and older) (del Carmen et al., 1999; Hoyo et al., 2005; Porterfield et al., 2003). Moreover, unlike newer screening procedures for other cancers, screening and treatment for CIN is generally covered by most insurance plans (Hoyo et al., 2005). Determining whether poorer access or a propensity for faster progressing lesions in African Americans would explain race/ethnic disparities is important, since eliminating disparities will depend on focusing limited resources to maximize access and/or to better understand the underlying mechanisms.

## 6.2 Cigarette Smoking

Since the first study that suggested an association between cervical cancer and cigarette smoking (Winkelstein, 1977), epidemiologic studies, including the largest study that pooled data from 23 studies with 13,541 cases and 23,017 controls, support evidence for an association between cigarette smoking and ICC, especially squamous cell carcinoma of the cervix (Appleby et al., 2006). In support of these findings, nicotine and cotinine have been found on cervical scrapes of women who smoke (Hellberg, Nilsson, Haley, Hoffman, & Wynder, 1988), leading to the interpretation that the mechanism may involve the accumulation of hydrophilic tobacco constituents on the cervix (Schiffman et al., 1993), which might favor CIN progression. In addition, a dose–response trend between number of pack-years of cigarettes smoked and lesion size was noted over a 6-month follow-up (Szarewski et al., 1996) and in relation to passive smoking (Trimble et al., 2005). A follow-up meta-analysis of CIN patients did not find an association between cigarette smoking and HPV clearance (Koshiol et al., 2006) or persistence (Harris et al., 2004; Syrjanen et al., 2007); however, an association with the cell proliferation marker *Ki67* was found (Harris et al., 2004), suggesting progression to CIN2+ associated with smoking may be independent of HPV. The prevalence of cigarette smoking is higher in European American women (Lee, Sobal, Frongillo, Olson, & Wolfe, 2005; Phares et al., 2004) than in African Americans, making differences in personal smoking an unlikely explanation of race/ethnic disparities in CIN2+ risk and ICC mortality, unless exposure to cigarette smoke can give rise to a more aggressive phenotype in African Americans.

## 6.3 Multiple Parity

Dose-dependent increase in the risk of ICC and CIS in relation to parity has been reported by some studies (Cuzick, Singer, De Stavola, & Chomet, 1990; Gupta et al., 2008; Hoyo et al., 2000, 2005; Munoz et al., 1993; Munoz, Castellsague, de Gonzalez, & Gissmann, 2006; Munoz et al., 2002), although other studies did not find this association (Becker, Wheeler, McGough, Stidley, et al., 1994). Cuzick et al. (1990) found that risk elevation—due to parity—trending upward existed only for CIS, but not CIN1 or CIN2. It has been reported that the prevalence of HPV16 and 18 infection increased as pregnancy progressed (Smith, Johnson, Jiang, & Zaleski, 1991), leading to the hypothesis that immune suppression, characteristic of pregnancy, may underlie the association between parity and ICC/CIS. Indeed a higher risk of ICC has been reported in women with lowered immune response, be it due to genetic predisposition (Stanczuk et al., 2001), iatrogenic, or otherwise acquired (Maiman et al., 1990; Schneider, 1993). In a 10-year follow-up study of CIN patients

(Castle et al., 2002), however, there was no evidence of an association between higher parity and progression to CIN3. Among parous women, parity is comparable in European American and African American women (Lee et al., 2005), and the recent increase in incidence of CIN lesions seen in developed countries is also not consistent with decreased fertility rates. This suggests that parity is unlikely to explain disparate CIN2+-related morbidity or mortality.

### 6.4 Oral Contraceptive Use

We and others, as well as meta-analyses involving 24 epidemiological studies with 16,573 cases and 35,509 controls, have reported an up to twofold increase in CIN2+ risk in women reporting oral contraceptive use, and the strength of this association increased with increasing duration of use (Beral, Hannaford, & Kay, 1988; Brinton et al., 1987; de Villiers, 2003; Gram, Macaluso, & Stalsberg, 1992; Hoyo et al., 2005; McFarlane-Anderson, Bazuaye, Jackson, Smikle, & Fletcher, 2008; Moreno et al., 2002; Munoz et al., 2002; Smith et al., 2003; Vanakankovit & Taneepanichskul, 2008). Others report no association (Castle et al., 2002; Green et al., 2003; Hoyo et al., 2005; La Vecchia et al., 1994; Thiry et al., 1993; Thomas & Ray, 1995) or an inverse association between oral contraceptive use and cervical dysplasia (Becker, Wheeler, McGough, Parmenter, et al., 1994). However, NHANES data suggest that oral contraceptive use is lower in African Americans than European Americans (Lee et al., 2005; Phares et al., 2004), suggesting that differences in the prevalence of hormonal contraceptive use are unlikely to account for race/ethnic differences observed in ICC and CIS incidence.

## 7. HPV GENETICS AND EPIGENETICS, AND ETHNIC DISPARITIES

DNA methylation in the viral genome allows many viruses to respond to environmental cues and regulate gene expression to evade the host immune system (Verma, 2003). HPV viral isolates that differ by <2% of the DNA sequence for the L1 gene are defined as variants, and this is true for any given HPV type. The L1 gene encodes the viral coat protein used as the antigen in the vaccines. HPV-type variants appear to segregate geographically (Wordlaw-Stinson et al., 2014) and to be race specific (American Cancer Society, 2005). Based on data from women with cytological interpretation of atypical cells of undetermined significance and those with low-grade lesions, it has been suggested that the distribution of HPV 16 and HPV 18 variants may be related to race among women presently living in the same geographic region (Xi et al., 2006). The European variants were more likely to persist in white women, while African variants were more likely to persist in African American women. Among white women, HPV 16 European variants were associated with a higher 2-year prevalence of CIN3 as compared to African American women (Xi et al., 2007). The *non-European* genetic variants within the long control region (LCR) of HPV16, 18, 52, and 33 have been consistently associated with a higher cross-sectional prevalence and higher risk of CIN persistence or progression (Formentin et al., 2013; Khouadri et al., 2006; Rodrigues-Coutlee et al., 2013; Sichero et al., 2007; Sichero, Franco, & Villa, 2005; Villa et al., 2000).

Data generated in the last decade also suggest that epigenetic modifications of the viral LCR (Badal et al., 2003; Piyathilake et al., 2011a, 2011b), the E5 (Bhattacharjee, Mandal, Roy, & Sengupta, 2008; Bhattacharjee & Sengupta, 2006), and E6 (Badal et al., 2003; Piyathilake et al., 2011a, 2014) genes of the most common HPV16 genotypes are associated with an altered trajectory for progression or risk of CIN2+. Given these data, HPV genetic and epigenetic variants have been proposed for inclusion into screening algorithms, to improve accuracy. However, these genetic and epigenetic variation data are available only for a handful of high-risk HPV genotypes including HPV 16, 18, 52, 45, and 33, yet data from several groups strongly suggest that the distributions of these genotypes vary by geography, SES, and race/ethnicity (Hariri et al., 2012; Khouadri et al., 2006; Niccolai et al., 2013; Vidal et al., 2011; Vidal, Smith, et al., 2014).

Emerging data also suggest that women who progress are often infected by more than one HPV genotype (Hariri et al., 2012; Niccolai et al., 2013; Vidal, Smith, et al., 2014), raising the possibility that progression could also be related to the sheer number, in addition to specific HPV genotypes. It has been hypothesized that the observed race-associated distribution of HPV variants may result from long-term sexual mixing patterns in the population or genetic influences of the host which preferentially predispose women to establish and/or retain infection with particular variants (Xi et al., 2013). While ethnic differences in the distribution of HPV genotypes and viral genetic differences may support that some of the ethnic or geographic variation could explain some disparities, the picture remains complex. Together these data raise the question of whether reducing disparities in cervical cancer incidence and mortality will require screening algorithms that include many more HPV genotypes, their genetics, and epigenetics.

## 8. HOST EPIGENETICS

Host epigenetic mechanisms have also been investigated and suggested to influence HPV infection predisposition, and progression to CIN and invasive cancer (Nye et al., 2013; Vidal, Henry, et al., 2014; Wisman et al., 2006). The effort put into identifying host-related biomarkers to distinguish cervical abnormalities likely to persist or progress from those likely to spontaneously regress has focused on host genetic (Frazer et al., 2006) and epigenetic (Wentzensen, Sherman, Schiffman, & Wang, 2009) factors. Stable epigenetic modifications contribute to the risk of progression (Feinberg, 2007a; Jirtle & Skinner, 2007). Because of the relative ease of measuring genomic DNA cytosine methylation at CpG dinucleotides, DNA methylation is the most commonly investigated epigenetic modification in epidemiologic studies. However, a review (Wentzensen et al., 2009) found that among studies evaluating up to 68 genes and ICC or CIN, only few had weak associations with DNA methylation levels at gene promoters or repeat elements. These regions have historically been targeted based on evidence that aberrant DNA methylation at promoter regions leads to transcriptional silencing, and loss of DNA methylation at *Alu* and *LINE* repeat elements occurs frequently in cancer where it is believed to result in chromosomal instability (Wilson, Power, & Molloy, 2007).

While informative, this narrow scope has precluded evaluation of numerous regulatory regions that are intragenic or intergenic (Wylie, Murphy, Orton, & Jirtle, 2000). Alternative replicable, cutting-edge approaches for selecting epigenetic targets include the agnostic genome-scale llumina Human 450K (Farkas, Milutin-Gasperov, Grce, & Nilsson, 2013; Huang et al., 2012) and DNA immunoprecipitation sequencing (MeDIP-Seq) covering ~2–40% of CpG sites within the genome. Supported by our preliminary data, these genome-scale approaches recently identified significant DNA methylation differences in promoter regions of *ZNF582, ZNF516,* and genomically imprinted *FKBP6* (Miyamato et al., 2006) and nonimprinted *CADM1* and *MAL* (Bierkens et al., 2013; De Vuyst et al., 2015) measured in DNA from tissue biopsies or exfoliated cervical cells of low- and high-grade squamous epithelial lesions (Brebi et al., 2014); this makes these loci promising candidates for identifying abnormal cytological findings likely to progress.

Candidate loci reported thus far are identified in case–control studies, yet the malleability of the methylation is still unknown. This temporal ambiguity had made their development into biomarkers difficult to justify. Moreover sample sizes are limited, and identified DNA methylation biomarkers lack corroborating mechanistic support. Importantly, the inherent tissue specificity of epigenetic marks may result in different DNA methylation marks in cervical tissues and exfoliated cervical cells. Exfoliated cervical cells are the most abundant cell type and frequently evaluated specimen in screening programs. Identifying methylation marks that predict progression to invasive cancer will require studies with wider and a deeper coverage of the epigenomic landscape. Also, the functional significance of regions identified will have to be demonstrated by either gene expression or the state of the chromatin.

## 8.1 Genomically Imprinted Genes Are Epigenetically Labile and Reasonable Candidates

Unlike other autosomal genes that are expressed from both the maternally and paternally derived chromosomal alleles, imprinted genes are expressed from only one allele while the other allele is transcriptionally silenced. The functional haploidy of these otherwise diploid genes makes them vulnerable to deregulation since a single genetic or epigenetic "hit" can completely abrogate gene function. Monoallelic gene expression is regulated by *cis*-acting DMRs (Carr, Yevtodiyenko, Schmidt, & Schmidt, 2007; Constancia, Pickard, Kelsey, & Reik, 1998; Delaval et al., 2007; Hu et al., 2000; Murphy & Jirtle, 2003; Reik & Walter, 2001; Vu, Jirtle, & Hoffman, 2006; Vu, Li, & Hoffman, 2004; Xin, Allis, & Wagstaff, 2001; Yang et al., 2003), and as such, aberrant methylation at these DMRs can disrupt normal patterns of gene expression and even the ability to maintain imprinted status. The methylation marks that regulate imprinted genes are somatically heritable, causing any alterations in methylation to be faithfully transmitted to daughter cells (Murphy et al., 2003). Haig's conflict hypothesis posits that imprinted genes are enriched for growth effectors that intricately interact to coordinate early growth, and coordinated control influences the expression of a "network" of imprinted genes throughout the genome (Haig, 1996a). To date, 156 human genes are predicted to be imprinted based on a bioinformatic approach (Luedi et al., 2007), and the imprinted status of 90 of these has been confirmed (Luedi et al., 2007).

## 8.2 Deregulation of Imprinted Genes and Human Malignancies

The growth regulatory role of imprinted genes emerges in deviant form in carcinogenesis where they are either aberrantly activated (Astuti et al., 2005; Cruz-Correa et al., 2004; Cui et al., 2003, 2001, 2002; Jelinic & Shaw, 2007; Kim, Choi, Niikawa, Lee, & Chang, 1998; Murphy et al., 2006; Oda, Shimizu, Minami, Kaneko, & Ishikawa, 1997; Rainho, Kowalski, & Rogatto, 2001; Ravenel et al., 2001; Sullivan, Taniguchi, Jhee, Kerr, & Reeve, 1999; Uyeno et al., 1996; van Roozendaal et al., 1998; Wu, Wang, et al., 1997; Wu, Weksberg, Minden, & Squire, 1997) or inactivated (Abdollahi et al., 2003; Kamikihara et al., 2005; Maegawa et al., 2001; Ng, Tang, Goh, & Hui, 2003; Yu et al., 2003, 1999; Yuan et al., 2003) through epigenetic mechanisms, presumably with consequent changes in the level of gene products produced. Arguably the best-studied imprinted gene in human cancer is *IGF2*, a paternally expressed gene that encodes a potent mitogenic growth factor that promotes cell proliferation (Chao & D'Amore, 2008; Hartmann et al., 2005). Increased expression of *IGF2* is often associated with loss of imprinting (LOI) where relaxation of imprint controls results in transcriptional activation of the normally silent maternal allele. In molecular studies, *IGF2* LOI is a frequent finding in Wilms' tumor (Rainier et al., 1993), hepatocellular carcinoma (Wu, Qin, Li, He, & Sun, 2008), bladder cancer (Byun et al., 2007), ovarian cancer (Kim et al., 1998; Murphy et al., 2006), and colon cancer (Cui et al., 2003, 2002; Nakagawa et al., 2001). Loss of *IGF2* imprinting was also found in 5 of 10 ICCs with no loss of heterozygosity (Douc-Rasy et al., 1996), although aberrant methylation at the intergenic *IGF2/H19* locus regulating *IGF2* was not evaluated. Inspection of microarray data from publically available data sets also suggests that *IGF2* is frequently overexpressed in invasive cancer. In support of these findings, a recent series of small ($n=20$) studies (Mathur et al., 2005) demonstrated an association between levels of protein encoded by *IGF2* and ICC as well as CIN. Spontaneous regression of the majority of these tumors was in consort with decreases in IGF2 protein levels. These protein levels were higher in women with high CIN grade and those with bulky tumors (>3 cm) compared to those with lower CIN grade or those with tumors <3 cm. When taken together, these studies provide a plausible mechanism for how deregulation of imprinted genes can contribute to progression from HPV infection to CIN2+.

Epigenetically induced increases in *IGF2* expression may alter the balance between progenitor and differentiated states in tissues, increasing the risk of proliferation. In a population-based, case–control study, a fivefold increase in risk of colorectal cancer was reported among individuals with LOI of *IGF2* in peripheral blood, and this correlated with LOI in colonic mucosa (Cruz-Correa et al., 2004). This association was confirmed by the same group (Cruz-Correa et al., 2004) and in another study where LOI was reported in normal colonic mucosa among individuals with colonic adenomas (Woodson et al., 2004). However, known risk factors for colorectal cancer including adulthood exposure to tobacco, alcohol, nonsteroidal antiinflammatory agents, and micronutrient intake (including folate, selenium, vitamins B6, B12, and B2), while associated with colorectal cancer, were not associated with risk of LOI in *IGF2*. This has led some (Feinberg, 2007b; Jirtle, 2004) to postulate that abnormal *IGF2* imprinting may not be acquired in adulthood, but rather, altered methylation that leads to LOI occurs in early life, during particular "windows of epigenetic vulnerability" when epigenetic reprogramming, rapid growth, and cell division may allow for environmentally induced epigenetic perturbations to be established. These findings imply that aberrant DNA methylation at growth regulatory loci may be informative for detecting earlier exposures, and identifying individuals that may be predisposed to progression to cervical cancer. This feature of imprinted genes should facilitate their use as stable "biosensors" of exposure that can be evaluated in case–control studies where exposures generally occur in the distant past, and as such are susceptible to recall bias.

## 8.3 Malleability of Aberrant Epigenetic Alterations

Since imprinted genes are regulated by epigenetic mechanisms, including DNA methylation, their expression patterns in part reflect the integrity, or lack there-of, of the epigenetic marks at their respective regulatory regions (Dean, Lucifero, & Santos, 2005; Hu et al., 2000; Ideraabdullah & Vigneau, 2008; Lewis et al., 2004; Yang et al., 2003). Emerging evidence suggests that although DNA methylation is a covalent modification, it is also malleable in response to environmental factors (Mathers, 2007), and this malleability provides public health intervention opportunities if exposures associated with deregulation are known. In mice, dietary shifts in the one-carbon metabolism pathway (the biochemical pathway that produces methyl group donors for cellular methylation reactions, including DNA methylation) altered methylation at several loci in the offspring, resulting in changes in gene expression and disease susceptibility (Waterland et al., 2006; Waterland & Jirtle, 2003). Postnatal methyl-deficient diets caused reversible changes in

*Igf2/H19* domain histone methylation and increased expression of both genes (Dobosy et al., 2008). Soy isoflavones were also found to increase methylation and expression of specific loci (Dolinoy, Weidman, Waterland, & Jirtle, 2006; Guerrero-Bosagna, Sabat, Valdovinos, Valladares, & Clark, 2008; Ho, Tang, Belmonte de Frausto, & Prins, 2006). Aberrant methylation alterations preceded cervical and vaginal cancer in the offspring exposed to diethylstilbestrol (Li et al., 2003) and vinclozolin (Anway, Cupp, Uzumcu, & Skinner, 2005; Anway, Leathers, & Skinner, 2006; Anway & Skinner, 2006). These data demonstrate that the epigenomic landscape is malleable postnatally. Exposures associated with aberrant methylation in humans in utero and postnatally are unknown and are an active topic of investigation by our group and others.

## 8.4 Imprinted Gene Networks and Potential Network Deregulation in Progression to Cancer

A fundamental characteristic of many imprinted genes is that they exist in gene clusters, primarily on human chromosomes 6, 7, 11, 14, and 15; higher order regulation of these clusters is thought to occur through the epigenetic marks present at imprinting centers (Lewis & Reik, 2006). The first evidence that imprinted genes are coordinately regulated came from studies of Beckwith–Wiedemann syndrome caused by defects in imprinting on chromosome 15 with affected individuals predisposed to Wilms' tumor and hepatoblastoma (Enklaar, Zabel, & Prawitt, 2006). Paternally expressed *ZAC* (aka *PLAGL1)* on chromosome 6 (Ma et al., 2004) encodes a DNA binding protein that functions as a tumor suppressor. ZAC binds in a methylation-sensitive manner to the nearby imprinted *LIT1* promoter CpG island that regulates expression of maternally expressed *CDKN1C* (aka $p57^{KIP2}$) on chromosome 15 in *cis* (Arima et al., 2005). Methylation of the *LIT1* promoter was found in several patients with transient neonatal diabetes along with altered expression/methylation of *ZAC*, suggesting that interaction between these two imprinted domains may contribute to this condition. These findings have led several investigators to propose that there is a more global methylation defect when imprint regulatory elements are epigenetically deregulated.

In mice, the realization that imprinted genes are coordinately regulated came from observations that there is coordinate downregulation concomitant with growth deceleration as somatic growth slows when approaching adult body size, a characteristic strongly supporting that these genes function together in a network (Lui, Finkielstain, Barnes, & Baron, 2008). The genes shown to exhibit coordinated repression with growth deceleration included *Igf2, H19, Zac, Mest, Peg3, Dlk1, Meg3, Grb10, Ndn, Cdkn1c*, and *SLC38a4*. In other mouse studies, *Zac* knockout disrupts a network of coordinately regulated genes that contain a large number that are imprinted. In vitro experiments showed induction of a number of imprinted genes on different chromosomes when *Zac* was overexpressed. Zac has also been shown to bind to the endodermal enhancers that drive paternal expression of *Igf2* and maternal expression of *H19*, and this binding trans-activates the promoters of both genes (Varrault et al., 2006). Evidence for an imprinted gene network is also supported by analysis of chromatin domains in other regions of the genome that interact with the *Igf2/H19* domain (Zhao et al., 2006). In this study, 114 domains were found to interact with the *Igf2/H19* domain, of which 21 of these were associated with 15 other imprinted genes.

Because imprinted genes are enriched for growth regulators and effectors (Haig, 2004) and they intricately interact to coordinate growth (Haig, 1996a, 1996b, 2000), when persistently dysregulated, they have the potential for widespread participation in cancer formation and progression (Feinberg, 2000, 2007a; Jirtle, 1999, 2004). Epigenetic dysregulation of these DMRs is an established feature of cancer initiation and progression (Cui et al., 2003; Feinberg, 2007a, 2007b). Published data support associations between aberrant DNA methylation at multiple other imprinted DMRs and CIN2+ or ICC (Nye et al., 2013; Vidal, Henry, et al., 2014), with the association between hypomethylation and ICC stronger than with CIN2/3. Nonetheless, patterns are difficult to discern with only a limited scope of DMRs evaluated and small sample sizes. It may take consortium arrangements to resolve these issues.

## 9. CONCLUDING REMARKS

Eliminating disparities in cervical cancer-related morbidity and mortality will require identification of markers that discriminate aggressive forms of CIN based on a more detailed understanding of progression from CIN1 to CIN2+. Current approaches are based on a combination of screening for HPV subtypes and putative cofactors. However, the distribution of *high-risk* and *intermediate*-risk HPV infection and cofactor patterns do not vary considerably by race/ethnicity to explain disparities in incidence and mortality related to CIN2+ observed in European Americans and African Americans, suggesting that inherent host response to these exposures underlies race/ethnic disparities in ICC. Epigenetic mechanisms contribute to CIN progression and can augment existing triage guidelines. However, a concerted effort is required to characterize the epigenomic landscape that together with HPV infection orchestrates progression from HPV infection to ICC.

## REFERENCES


Abdollahi, A., Pisarcik, D., Roberts, D., Weinstein, J., Cairns, P., & Hamilton, T. C. (2003). LOT1 (PLAGL1/ZAC1), the candidate tumor suppressor gene at chromosome 6q24-25, is epigenetically regulated in cancer. *The Journal of Biological Chemistry*, *278*(8), 6041–6049.

Akers, A. Y., Newmann, S. J., & Smith, J. S. (2007). Factors underlying disparities in cervical cancer incidence, screening, and treatment in the United States. *Current Problems in Cancer*, *31*(3), 157–181.

American Cancer Society. (2005). Cancer facts & figures for African Americans 2005-2006. In American Cancer Society (Ed.), *Cancer facts & figures* (p. 24). Atlanta, GA: American Cancer Society.

American Cancer Society. (2012). Cancer facts and figures 2012. In American Cancer Society (Ed.), *Cancer facts and figures*. Atlanta, GA: American Cancer Society.

Anway, M. D., Cupp, A. S., Uzumcu, M., & Skinner, M. K. (2005). Epigenetic transgenerational actions of endocrine disruptors and male fertility. *Science (New York, N.Y.)*, *308*(5727), 1466–1469.

Anway, M. D., Leathers, C., & Skinner, M. K. (2006). Endocrine disruptor vinclozolin induced epigenetic transgenerational adult onset disease. *Endocrinology*, *147*(12), 5512–5523.

Anway, M. D., & Skinner, M. K. (2006). Epigenetic transgenerational actions of endocrine disruptors. *Endocrinology*, *147*(6 Suppl.), S43–S49.

Appleby, P., Beral, V., Berrington de Gonzalez, A., Colin, D., Franceschi, S., Goodill, A., et al. (2006). Carcinoma of the cervix and tobacco smoking: Collaborative reanalysis of individual data on 13,541 women with carcinoma of the cervix and 23,017 women without carcinoma of the cervix from 23 epidemiological studies. *International Journal of Cancer*, *118*(6), 1481–1495.

Arends, M. J., Buckley, C. H., & Wells, M. (1998). Aetiology, pathogenesis, and pathology of cervical neoplasia. *Journal of Clinical Pathology*, *51*(2), 96–103.

Arima, T., Kamikihara, T., Hayashida, T., Kato, K., Inoue, T., Shirayoshi, Y., et al. (2005). ZAC, LIT1 (KCNQ1OT1) and p57KIP2 (CDKN1C) are in an imprinted gene network that may play a role in Beckwith-Wiedemann syndrome. *Nucleic Acids Research*, *33*(8), 2650–2660.

Astuti, D., Latif, F., Wagner, K., Gentle, D., Cooper, W. N., Catchpoole, D., et al. (2005). Epigenetic alteration at the DLK1-GTL2 imprinted domain in human neoplasia: Analysis of neuroblastoma, phaeochromocytoma and Wilms' tumour. *British Journal of Cancer*, *92*(8), 1574–1580.

Badal, V., Chuang, L. S., Tan, E. H., Badal, S., Villa, L. L., Wheeler, C. M., et al. (2003). CpG methylation of human papillomavirus type 16 DNA in cervical cancer cell lines and in clinical specimens: Genomic hypomethylation correlates with carcinogenic progression. *Journal of Virology*, 77(11), 6227–6234.

Becker, T. M., Wheeler, C. M., McGough, N. S., Jordan, S. W., Dorin, M., & Miller, J. (1991). Cervical papillomavirus infection and cervical dysplasia in Hispanic, Native American, and non-Hispanic white women in New Mexico. *American Journal of Public Health*, *81*(5), 582–586.

Becker, T. M., Wheeler, C. M., McGough, N. S., Parmenter, C. A., Jordan, S. W., Stidley, C. A., et al. (1994). Sexually transmitted diseases and other risk factors for cervical dysplasia among southwestern Hispanic and non-Hispanic white women. *JAMA, 271*(15), 1181–1188.

Becker, T. M., Wheeler, C. M., McGough, N. S., Stidley, C. A., Parmenter, C. A., Dorin, M., et al. (1994). Contraceptive and reproductive risks for cervical dysplasia in southwestern Hispanic and non-Hispanic white women. *International Journal of Epidemiology, 23*(5), 913–922.

Beral, V., Hannaford, P., & Kay, C. (1988). Oral contraceptive use and malignancies of the genital tract. Results from the Royal College of General Practitioners' Oral Contraception Study. *Lancet, 2*(8624), 1331–1335.

Bhattacharjee, B., Mandal, N. R., Roy, S., & Sengupta, S. (2008). Characterization of sequence variations within HPV16 isolates among Indian women: Prediction of causal role of rare non-synonymous variations within intact isolates in cervical cancer pathogenesis. *Virology, 377*(1), 143–150.

Bhattacharjee, B., & Sengupta, S. (2006). HPV16 E2 gene disruption and polymorphisms of E2 and LCR: Some significant associations with cervical cancer in Indian women. *Gynecologic Oncology, 100*(2), 372–378.

Bierkens, M., Hesselink, A. T., Meijer, C. J., Heideman, D. A., Wisman, G. B., van der Zee, A. G., et al. (2013). CADM1 and MAL promoter methylation levels in hrHPV-positive cervical scrapes increase proportional to degree and duration of underlying cervical disease. *International Journal of Cancer, 133*(6), 1293–1299.

Bosch, F. X., Munoz, N., de Sanjose, S., Navarro, C., Moreo, P., Ascunce, N., et al. (1993). Human papillomavirus and cervical intraepithelial neoplasia grade III/carcinoma in situ: A case-control study in Spain and Colombia. *Cancer Epidemiology, Biomarkers & Prevention, 2*(5), 415–422.

Brebi, P., Maldonado, L., Noordhuis, M. G., Ili, C., Leal, P., Garcia, P., et al. (2014). Genome-wide methylation profiling reveals Zinc finger protein 516 (ZNF516) and FK-506-binding protein 6 (FKBP6) promoters frequently methylated in cervical neoplasia, associated with HPV status and ethnicity in a Chilean population. *Epigenetics, 9*(2), 308–317.

Brinton, L. A., Tashima, K. T., Lehman, H. F., Levine, R. S., Mallin, K., Savitz, D. A., et al. (1987). Epidemiology of cervical cancer by cell type. *Cancer Research, 47*(6), 1706–1711.

Byun, H. M., Wong, H. L., Birnstein, E. A., Wolff, E. M., Liang, G., & Yang, A. S. (2007). Examination of IGF2 and H19 loss of imprinting in bladder cancer. *Cancer Research, 67*(22), 10753–10758.

Carr, M. S., Yevtodiyenko, A., Schmidt, C. L., & Schmidt, J. V. (2007). Allele-specific histone modifications regulate expression of the Dlk1-Gtl2 imprinted domain. *Genomics, 89*(2), 280–290.

Castle, P. E., Wacholder, S., Lorincz, A. T., Scott, D. R., Sherman, M. E., Glass, A. G., et al. (2002). A prospective study of high-grade cervical neoplasia risk among human papillomavirus-infected women. *Journal of the National Cancer Institute, 94*(18), 1406–1414.

Chan, P. G., Sung, H. Y., & Sawaya, G. F. (2003). Changes in cervical cancer incidence after three decades of screening US women less than 30 years old. *Obstetrics and Gynecology, 102*(4), 765–773.

Chao, W., & D'Amore, P. A. (2008). IGF2: Epigenetic regulation and role in development and disease. *Cytokine & Growth Factor Reviews, 19*(2), 111–120.

Choo, K. B., Pan, C. C., Liu, M. S., Ng, H. T., Chen, C. P., Lee, Y. N., et al. (1987). Presence of episomal and integrated human papillomavirus DNA sequences in cervical carcinoma. *Journal of Medical Virology, 21*(2), 101–107.

Chumworathayi, B., Eamratsameekool, W., Kularbkaew, C., & Chumworathayi, P. (2008). Visual inspection with acetic acid test qualities in a secondary setting. *The Journal of Obstetrics and Gynaecology Research, 34*(5), 909–913.

Coker, A. L., Jenkins, G. R., Busnardo, M. S., Chambers, J. C., Levine, L. Z., & Pirisi, L. (1993). Human papillomaviruses and cervical neoplasia in South Carolina. *Cancer Epidemiology, Biomarkers & Prevention, 2*(3), 207–212.

Constancia, M., Pickard, B., Kelsey, G., & Reik, W. (1998). Imprinting mechanisms. *Genome Research, 8*(9), 881–900.

Cortecchia, S., Galanti, G., Sgadari, C., Costa, S., De Lillo, M., Caprara, L., et al. (2013). Follow-up study of patients with cervical intraepithelial neoplasia grade 1 overexpressing p16Ink4a. *International Journal of Gynecological Cancer, 23*(9), 1663–1669.

Cruz-Correa, M., Cui, H., Giardiello, F. M., Powe, N. R., Hylind, L., Robinson, A., et al. (2004). Loss of imprinting of insulin growth factor II gene: A potential heritable biomarker for colon neoplasia predisposition. *Gastroenterology, 126*(4), 964–970.

Cui, H., Cruz-Correa, M., Giardiello, F. M., Hutcheon, D. F., Kafonek, D. R., Brandenburg, S., et al. (2003). Loss of IGF2 imprinting: A potential marker of colorectal cancer risk. *Science (New York, N.Y.), 299*(5613), 1753–1755.

Cui, H., Niemitz, E. L., Ravenel, J. D., Onyango, P., Brandenburg, S. A., Lobanenkov, V. V., et al. (2001). Loss of imprinting of insulin-like growth factor-II in Wilms' tumor commonly involves altered methylation but not mutations of CTCF or its binding site. *Cancer Research, 61*(13), 4947–4950.

Cui, H., Onyango, P., Brandenburg, S., Wu, Y., Hsieh, C. L., & Feinberg, A. P. (2002). Loss of imprinting in colorectal cancer linked to hypomethylation of H19 and IGF2. *Cancer Research, 62*(22), 6442–6446.

Cuzick, J., Singer, A., De Stavola, B. L., & Chomet, J. (1990). Case-control study of risk factors for cervical intraepithelial neoplasia in young women. *European Journal of Cancer, 26*(6), 684–690.

de Villiers, E. M. (2003). Relationship between steroid hormone contraceptives and HPV, cervical intraepithelial neoplasia and cervical carcinoma. *International Journal of Cancer, 103*(6), 705–708.

De Vuyst, H., Franceschi, S., Plummer, M., Mugo, N. R., Sakr, S. R., Meijer, C. J., et al. (2015). Methylation levels of CADM1, MAL, and MIR124-2 in cervical scrapes for triage of HIV-infected, high-risk HPV-positive women in Kenya. *Journal of Acquired Immune Deficiency Syndromes, 70*(3), 311–318.

Dean, W., Lucifero, D., & Santos, F. (2005). DNA methylation in mammalian development and disease. *Birth Defects Research. Part C, Embryo Today, 75*(2), 98–111.

del Carmen, M. G., Montz, F. J., Bristow, R. E., Bovicelli, A., Cornelison, T., & Trimble, E. (1999). Ethnic differences in patterns of care of stage 1A(1) and stage 1A(2) cervical cancer: A SEER database study. *Gynecologic Oncology, 75*(1), 113–117.

del Pino, M., Garcia, S., Fuste, V., Alonso, I., Fuste, P., Torne, A., et al. (2009). Value of p16 (INK4a) as a marker of progression/regression in cervical intraepithelial neoplasia grade 1. *American Journal of Obstetrics and Gynecology, 201*(5), 488.e481–488.e487.

Delaval, K., Govin, J., Cerqueira, F., Rousseaux, S., Khochbin, S., & Feil, R. (2007). Differential histone modifications mark mouse imprinting control regions during spermatogenesis. *The EMBO Journal, 26*(3), 720–729.

Dobosy, J. R., Fu, V. X., Desotelle, J. A., Srinivasan, R., Kenowski, M. L., Almassi, N., et al. (2008). A methyl-deficient diet modifies histone methylation and alters Igf2 and H19 repression in the prostate. *Prostate, 68*(11), 1187–1195.

Dolinoy, D. C., Weidman, J. R., Waterland, R. A., & Jirtle, R. L. (2006). Maternal genistein alters coat color and protects Avy mouse offspring from obesity by modifying the fetal epigenome. *Environmental Health Perspectives, 114*(4), 567–572.

Douc-Rasy, S., Barrois, M., Fogel, S., Ahomadegbe, J. C., Stehelin, D., Coll, J., et al. (1996). High incidence of loss of heterozygosity and abnormal imprinting of H19 and IGF2 genes in invasive cervical carcinomas. Uncoupling of H19 and IGF2 expression and biallelic hypomethylation of H19. *Oncogene*, *12*(2), 423–430.

Dunne, E. F., Unger, E. R., Sternberg, M., McQuillan, G., Swan, D. C., Patel, S. S., et al. (2007). Prevalence of HPV infection among females in the United States. *JAMA*, *297*(8), 813–819.

Eggleston, K. S., Coker, A. L., Luchok, K. J., & Meyer, T. E. (2007). Adherence to recommendations for follow-up to abnormal Pap tests. *Obstetrics and Gynecology*, *109*(6), 1332–1341.

Enklaar, T., Zabel, B. U., & Prawitt, D. (2006). Beckwith-Wiedemann syndrome: Multiple molecular mechanisms. *Expert Reviews in Molecular Medicine*, *8*(17), 1–19.

Farkas, S. A., Milutin-Gasperov, N., Grce, M., & Nilsson, T. K. (2013). Genome-wide DNA methylation assay reveals novel candidate biomarker genes in cervical cancer. *Epigenetics*, *8*(11), 1213–1225.

Farley, J. H., Hines, J. F., Taylor, R. R., Carlson, J. W., Parker, M. F., Kost, E. R., et al. (2001). Equal care ensures equal survival for African-American women with cervical carcinoma. *Cancer*, *91*(4), 869–873.

Feinberg, A. P. (2000). DNA methylation, genomic imprinting and cancer. *Current Topics in Microbiology and Immunology*, *249*, 87–99.

Feinberg, A. P. (2007a). Phenotypic plasticity and the epigenetics of human disease. *Nature*, *447*(7143), 433–440.

Feinberg, A. P. (2007b). An epigenetic approach to cancer etiology. *Cancer Journal (Sudbury Mass.)*, *13*(1), 70–74.

Ferris, D. G., Waller, J. L., Owen, A., & Smith, J. (2007). Midadult women's attitudes about receiving the prophylactic human papillomavirus vaccine. *Journal of Lower Genital Tract Disease*, *11*(3), 166–172.

Formentin, A., Archambault, J., Koushik, A., Richardson, H., Brassard, P., Franco, E. L., et al. (2013). Human papillomavirus type 52 polymorphism and high-grade lesions of the uterine cervix. *International Journal of Cancer*, *132*(8), 1821–1830.

Franco, E. L. (2003). Chapter 13: Primary screening of cervical cancer with human papillomavirus tests. *Journal of the National Cancer Institute. Monographs*, *31*, 89–96.

Franco, E. L., Duarte-Franco, E., & Ferenczy, A. (2001). Cervical cancer: Epidemiology, prevention and the role of human papillomavirus infection. *CMAJ*, *164*(7), 1017–1025.

Franco, E. L., & Ferenczy, A. (2002). Cervix. In E. L. Franco & T. E. Rohan (Eds.), *Cancer precursors: Epidemiology, detection, and prevention*. New York: Springer-Verlag.

Franco, E. L., Schlecht, N. F., & Saslow, D. (2003). The epidemiology of cervical cancer. *Cancer Journal (Sudbury Mass.)*, *9*(5), 348–359.

Frazer, I. H., Cox, J. T., Mayeaux, E. J., Jr., Franco, E. L., Moscicki, A. B., Palefsky, J. M., et al. (2006). Advances in prevention of cervical cancer and other human papillomavirus-related diseases. *The Pediatric Infectious Disease Journal*, *25*(2 Suppl.), S65–S81. quiz S82.

Goldstein, B. Y., Bray, F. I., Parkin, D. M., Sellors, J. W., & Zhang, Z. F. (2010). *Years of life lost from lung, stomach, liver and cervical cancers: An evaluation of the top cancer killers. Handbook of disease burdens and quality of life measures*. New York: Springer, pp. 825–842.

Gram, I. T., Macaluso, M., & Stalsberg, H. (1992). Oral contraceptive use and the incidence of cervical intraepithelial neoplasia. *American Journal of Obstetrics and Gynecology*, *167*(1), 40–44.

Green, J., Berrington de Gonzalez, A., Sweetland, S., Beral, V., Chilvers, C., Crossley, B., et al. (2003). Risk factors for adenocarcinoma and squamous cell carcinoma of the cervix in women aged 20-44 years: The UK National Case-Control Study of Cervical Cancer. *British Journal of Cancer*, *89*(11), 2078–2086.

Guerrero-Bosagna, C. M., Sabat, P., Valdovinos, F. S., Valladares, L. E., & Clark, S. J. (2008). Epigenetic and phenotypic changes result from a continuous pre and post natal dietary exposure to phytoestrogens in an experimental population of mice. *BMC Physiology*, *8*, 17.

Gupta, S., Sodhani, P., Sharma, A., Sharma, J. K., Halder, K., Charchra, K. L., et al. (2008). Prevalence of high-risk human papillomavirus type 16/18 infection among women with normal cytology: Risk factor analysis and implications for screening and prophylaxis. *Cytopathology*, *20*, 249–255.

Haig, D. (1996a). Do imprinted genes have few and small introns? *Bioessays*, *18*(5), 351–353.

Haig, D. (1996b). Altercation of generations: Genetic conflicts of pregnancy. *American Journal of Reproductive Immunology*, *35*(3), 226–232.

Haig, D. (2000). Genomic imprinting, sex-biased dispersal, and social behavior. *Annals of the New York Academy of Sciences*, *907*, 149–163.

Haig, D. (2004). Genomic imprinting and kinship: How good is the evidence? *Annual Review of Genetics*, *38*, 553–585.

Hariri, S., Johnson, M. L., Bennett, N. M., Bauer, H. M., Park, I. U., Schafer, S., et al. (2015). Population-based trends in high-grade cervical lesions in the early human papillomavirus vaccine era in the United States. *Cancer*, *121*(16), 2775–2781.

Hariri, J., & Oster, A. (2007). The negative predictive value of p16INK4a to assess the outcome of cervical intraepithelial neoplasia 1 in the uterine cervix. *International Journal of Gynecological Pathology*, *26*(3), 223–228.

Hariri, S., Unger, E. R., Powell, S. E., Bauer, H. M., Bennett, N. M., Bloch, K. C., et al. (2012). Human papillomavirus genotypes in high-grade cervical lesions in the United States. *The Journal of Infectious Diseases*, *206*(12), 1878–1886.

Harris, T. G., Kulasingam, S. L., Kiviat, N. B., Mao, C., Agoff, S. N., Feng, Q., et al. (2004). Cigarette smoking, oncogenic human papillomavirus, Ki-67 antigen, and cervical intraepithelial neoplasia. *American Journal of Epidemiology*, *159*(9), 834–842.

Hartmann, W., Koch, A., Brune, H., Waha, A., Schuller, U., Dani, I., et al. (2005). Insulin-like growth factor II is involved in the proliferation control of medulloblastoma and its cerebellar precursor cells. *The American Journal of Pathology*, *166*(4), 1153–1162.

Hellberg, D., Nilsson, S., Haley, N. J., Hoffman, D., & Wynder, E. (1988). Smoking and cervical intraepithelial neoplasia: Nicotine and cotinine in serum and cervical mucus in smokers and nonsmokers. *American Journal of Obstetrics and Gynecology*, *158*(4), 910–913.

Hernandez, B. Y., McDuffie, K., Franke, A. A., Killeen, J., & Goodman, M. T. (2004). Reports: Plasma and dietary phytoestrogens and risk of premalignant lesions of the cervix. *Nutrition and Cancer*, *49*(2), 109–124.

Ho, S. M., Tang, W. Y., Belmonte de Frausto, J., & Prins, G. S. (2006). Developmental exposure to estradiol and bisphenol A increases susceptibility to prostate carcinogenesis and epigenetically regulates phosphodiesterase type 4 variant 4. *Cancer Research*, *66*(11), 5624–5632.

Hoyo, C., Miller, W. C., Newman, B. M., & Fortney, J. A. (2000). Selective screening for cervical neoplasia: An approach for resource-poor settings. *International Journal of Epidemiology*, *29*(5), 807–812.

Hoyo, C., Yarnall, K. S., Skinner, C. S., Moorman, P. G., Sellers, D., & Reid, L. (2005). Pain predicts non-adherence to pap smear screening among middle-aged African American women. *Preventive Medicine*, *41*(2), 439–445.

Hu, J. F., Pham, J., Dey, I., Li, T., Vu, T. H., & Hoffman, A. R. (2000). Allele-specific histone acetylation accompanies genomic imprinting of the insulin-like growth factor II receptor gene. *Endocrinology*, *141*(12), 4428–4435.

Huang, R. L., Chang, C. C., Su, P. H., Chen, Y. C., Liao, Y. P., Wang, H. C., et al. (2012). Methylomic analysis identifies frequent DNA methylation of zinc finger protein 582 (ZNF582) in cervical neoplasms. *PLoS One*, 7(7), e41060.

Ideraabdullah, F. Y., & Vigneau, S. (2008). Genomic imprinting mechanisms in mammals. *Mutation Research*, *647*, 77–85.

Jelinic, P., & Shaw, P. (2007). Loss of imprinting and cancer. *The Journal of Pathology*, *211*(3), 261–268.

Jemal, A., Bray, F., Center, M. M., Ferlay, J., Ward, E., & Forman, D. (2011). Global cancer statistics. *CA: A Cancer Journal for Clinicians*, *61*(2), 69–90.

Jirtle, R. L. (1999). Genomic imprinting and cancer. *Experimental Cell Research*, *248*(1), 18–24.

Jirtle, R. L. (2004). IGF2 loss of imprinting: A potential heritable risk factor for colorectal cancer. *Gastroenterology*, *126*(4), 1190–1193.

Jirtle, R. L. (2009). Epigenome: The program for human health and disease. *Epigenomics*, *1*(1), 13–15.

Jirtle, R. L., & Skinner, M. K. (2007). Environmental epigenomics and disease susceptibility. *Nature Reviews. Genetics*, *8*(4), 253–262.

Kadish, A. S., Hagan, R. J., Ritter, D. B., Goldberg, G. L., Romney, S. L., Kanetsky, P. A., et al. (1992). Biologic characteristics of specific human papillomavirus types predicted from morphology of cervical lesions. *Human Pathology*, *23*(11), 1262–1269.

Kahn, J. A., Lan, D., & Kahn, R. S. (2007). Sociodemographic factors associated with high-risk human papillomavirus infection. *Obstetrics and Gynecology*, *110*(1), 87–95.

Kamikihara, T., Arima, T., Kato, K., Matsuda, T., Kato, H., Douchi, T., et al. (2005). Epigenetic silencing of the imprinted gene ZAC by DNA methylation is an early event in the progression of human ovarian cancer. *International Journal of Cancer*, *115*(5), 690–700.

Khouadri, S., Villa, L. L., Gagnon, S., Koushik, A., Richardson, H., Ferreira, S., et al. (2006). Human papillomavirus type 33 polymorphisms and high-grade squamous intraepithelial lesions of the uterine cervix. *The Journal of Infectious Diseases*, *194*(7), 886–894.

Kim, H. T., Choi, B. H., Niikawa, N., Lee, T. S., & Chang, S. I. (1998). Frequent loss of imprinting of the H19 and IGF-II genes in ovarian tumors. *American Journal of Medical Genetics*, *80*(4), 391–395.

Koshiol, J., Schroeder, J., Jamieson, D. J., Marshall, S. W., Duerr, A., Heilig, C. M., et al. (2006). Smoking and time to clearance of human papillomavirus infection in HIV-seropositive and HIV-seronegative women. *American Journal of Epidemiology*, *164*(2), 176–183.

Koutsky, L. A., Holmes, K. K., Critchlow, C. W., Stevens, C. E., Paavonen, J., Beckmann, A. M., et al. (1992). A cohort study of the risk of cervical intraepithelial neoplasia grade 2 or 3 in relation to papillomavirus infection. *The New England Journal of Medicine*, *327*(18), 1272–1278.

La Vecchia, C., D'Avanzo, B., Franceschi, S., Negri, E., Parazzini, F., & Decarli, A. (1994). Menstrual and reproductive factors and gastric-cancer risk in women. *International Journal of Cancer*, *59*(6), 761–764.

Lee, S. K., Sobal, J., Frongillo, E. A., Olson, C. M., & Wolfe, W. S. (2005). Parity and body weight in the United States: Differences by race and size of place of residence. *Obesity Research*, *13*(7), 1263–1269.

Levine, A. J., Harper, J., Hilborne, L., Rosenthal, D. L., Weismeier, E., & Haile, R. W. (1993). HPV DNA and the risk of squamous intraepithelial lesions of the uterine cervix in young women. *American Journal of Clinical Pathology*, *100*(1), 6–11.

Lewis, A., Mitsuya, K., Umlauf, D., Smith, P., Dean, W., Walter, J., et al. (2004). Imprinting on distal chromosome 7 in the placenta involves repressive histone methylation independent of DNA methylation. *Nature Genetics*, *36*(12), 1291–1295.

Lewis, A., & Reik, W. (2006). How imprinting centres work. *Cytogenetic and Genome Research*, *113*(1–4), 81–89.

Li, S., Hansman, R., Newbold, R., Davis, B., McLachlan, J. A., & Barrett, J. C. (2003). Neonatal diethylstilbestrol exposure induces persistent elevation of c-fos expression and hypomethylation in its exon-4 in mouse uterus. *Molecular Carcinogenesis*, *38*(2), 78–84.

Liao, G. D., Sellors, J. W., Sun, H. K., Zhang, X., Bao, Y. P., Jeronimo, J., et al. (2014). p16INK4A immunohistochemical staining and predictive value for progression of cervical intraepithelial neoplasia grade 1: A prospective study in China. *International Journal of Cancer, 134*(7), 1715–1724.
Luedi, P. P., Dietrich, F. S., Weidman, J. R., Bosko, J. M., Jirtle, R. L., & Hartemink, A. J. (2007). Computational and experimental identification of novel human imprinted genes. *Genome Research, 17*(12), 1723–1730.
Lui, J. C., Finkielstain, G. P., Barnes, K. M., & Baron, J. (2008). An imprinted gene network that controls mammalian somatic growth is down-regulated during postnatal growth deceleration in multiple organs. *American Journal of Physiology, 30*, 30.
Ma, D., Shield, J. P., Dean, W., Leclerc, I., Knauf, C., Burcelin, R. R., et al. (2004). Impaired glucose homeostasis in transgenic mice expressing the human transient neonatal diabetes mellitus locus, TNDM. *The Journal of Clinical Investigation, 114*(3), 339–348.
Maegawa, S., Yoshioka, H., Itaba, N., Kubota, N., Nishihara, S., Shirayoshi, Y., et al. (2001). Epigenetic silencing of PEG3 gene expression in human glioma cell lines. *Molecular Carcinogenesis, 31*(1), 1–9.
Maiman, M., Fruchter, R. G., Serur, E., Remy, J. C., Feuer, G., & Boyce, J. (1990). Human immunodeficiency virus infection and cervical neoplasia. *Gynecologic Oncology, 38*(3), 377–382.
Markowitz, L. E., Liu, G., Hariri, S., Steinau, M., Dunne, E. F., & Unger, E. R. (2016). Prevalence of HPV after introduction of the vaccination program in the United States. *Pediatrics, 137*(3), e20151968.
Mathers, J. C. (2007). Early nutrition: Impact on epigenetics. *Forum of Nutrition, 60*, 42–48.
Mathur, S. P., Mathur, R. S., Gray, E. A., Lane, D., Underwood, P. G., Kohler, M., et al. (2005). Serum vascular endothelial growth factor C (VEGF-C) as a specific biomarker for advanced cervical cancer: Relationship to insulin-like growth factor II (IGF-II), IGF binding protein 3 (IGF-BP3) and VEGF-A [corrected]. *Gynecologic Oncology, 98*(3), 467–483.
McFarlane-Anderson, N., Bazuaye, P. E., Jackson, M. D., Smikle, M., & Fletcher, H. M. (2008). Cervical dysplasia and cancer and the use of hormonal contraceptives in Jamaican women. *BMC Women's Health, 8*, 9.
Mills, A. M., Paquette, C., Castle, P. E., & Stoler, M. H. (2015). Risk stratification by p16 immunostaining of CIN1 biopsies: A retrospective study of patients from the quadrivalent HPV vaccine trials. *The American Journal of Surgical Pathology, 39*(5), 611–617.
Miyamato, T., Sato, H., Yogev, L., Kleiman, S., Namiki, M., Koh, E., et al. (2006). Is a genetic defect in Fkbp6 a common cause of azoospermia in humans? *Cellular & Molecular Biology Letters, 11*(4), 557–569.
Moreno, V., Bosch, F. X., Munoz, N., Meijer, C. J., Shah, K. V., Walboomers, J. M., et al. (2002). Effect of oral contraceptives on risk of cervical cancer in women with human papillomavirus infection: The IARC multicentric case-control study. *Lancet, 359*(9312), 1085–1092.
Morrison, E. A., Ho, G. Y., Vermund, S. H., Goldberg, G. L., Kadish, A. S., Kelley, K. F., et al. (1991). Human papillomavirus infection and other risk factors for cervical neoplasia: A case-control study. *International Journal of Cancer, 49*(1), 6–13.
Munoz, N., Bosch, F. X., de Sanjose, S., Vergara, A., del Moral, A., Munoz, M. T., et al. (1993). Risk factors for cervical intraepithelial neoplasia grade III/carcinoma in situ in Spain and Colombia. *Cancer Epidemiology, Biomarkers & Prevention, 2*(5), 423–431.
Munoz, N., Castellsague, X., de Gonzalez, A. B., & Gissmann, L. (2006). Chapter 1: HPV in the etiology of human cancer. *Vaccine, 24*(Suppl. 3). S3/1–S3/10.
Munoz, N., Franceschi, S., Bosetti, C., Moreno, V., Herrero, R., Smith, J. S., et al. (2002). Role of parity and human papillomavirus in cervical cancer: The IARC multicentric case-control study. *Lancet, 359*(9312), 1093–1101.

Murphy, S. K., Huang, Z., Wen, Y., Spillman, M. A., Whitaker, R. S., Simel, L. R., et al. (2006). Frequent IGF2/H19 domain epigenetic alterations and elevated IGF2 expression in epithelial ovarian cancer. *Molecular Cancer Research*, *4*(4), 283–292.

Murphy, S. K., & Jirtle, R. L. (2003). Imprinting evolution and the price of silence. *Bioessays*, *25*(6), 577–588.

Murphy, S. K., Wylie, A. A., Coveler, K. J., Cotter, P. D., Papenhausen, P. R., Sutton, V. R., et al. (2003). Epigenetic detection of human chromosome 14 uniparental disomy. *Human Mutation*, *22*(1), 92–97.

Nakagawa, H. H., Chadwick, R. R. B., Peltomaki, P. P., Plass, C. C., Nakamura, Y. Y., & de La Chapelle, A. A. (2001). Loss of imprinting of the insulin-like growth factor II gene occurs by biallelic methylation in a core region of H19-associated CTCF-binding sites in colorectal cancer. *Proceedings of the National Academy of Sciences of the United States of America*, *98*(2), 591–596.

Ng, A., Tang, J. P., Goh, C. H., & Hui, K. M. (2003). Regulation of the H19 imprinting gene expression in human nasopharyngeal carcinoma by methylation. *International Journal of Cancer*, *104*(2), 179–187.

Niccolai, L. M., Russ, C., Julian, P. J., Hariri, S., Sinard, J., Meek, J. I., et al. (2013). Individual and geographic disparities in human papillomavirus types 16/18 in high-grade cervical lesions: Associations with race, ethnicity, and poverty. *Cancer*, *119*(16), 3052–3058.

Nye, M. D., Hoyo, C., Huang, Z., Vidal, A. C., Wang, F., Overcash, F., et al. (2013). Associations between methylation of paternally expressed gene 3 (PEG3), cervical intraepithelial neoplasia and invasive cervical cancer. *PLoS One*, *8*(2), e56325.

Oda, H., Shimizu, S., Minami, K., Kaneko, K., & Ishikawa, T. (1997). Loss of imprinting of the IGF2 gene in a Wilms' tumor in an adult. *Journal of the National Cancer Institute*, *89*(23), 1813–1814.

Ozaki, S., Zen, Y., & Inoue, M. (2011). Biomarker expression in cervical intraepithelial neoplasia: Potential progression predictive factors for low-grade lesions. *Human Pathology*, *42*(7), 1007–1012.

Pacchiarotti, A., Ferrari, F., Bellardini, P., Chini, F., Collina, G., Dalla Palma, P., et al. (2014). Prognostic value of p16-INK4A protein in women with negative or CIN1 histology result: A follow-up study. *International Journal of Cancer*, *134*(4), 897–904.

Phares, T. M., Morrow, B., Lansky, A., Barfield, W. D., Prince, C. B., Marchi, K. S., et al. (2004). Surveillance for disparities in maternal health-related behaviors—Selected states, Pregnancy Risk Assessment Monitoring System (PRAMS), 2000-2001. *MMWR Surveillance Summaries*, *53*(4), 1–13.

Piyathilake, C. J., Macaluso, M., Alvarez, R. D., Chen, M., Badiga, S., Edberg, J. C., et al. (2011a). A higher degree of methylation of the HPV 16 E6 gene is associated with a lower likelihood of being diagnosed with cervical intraepithelial neoplasia. *Cancer*, *117*(5), 957–963.

Piyathilake, C. J., Macaluso, M., Alvarez, R. D., Chen, M., Badiga, S., Siddiqui, N. R., et al. (2011b). A higher degree of LINE-1 methylation in peripheral blood mononuclear cells, a one-carbon nutrient related epigenetic alteration, is associated with a lower risk of developing cervical intraepithelial neoplasia. *Nutrition (Burbank, Los Angeles County, Calif.)*, *27*(5), 513–519.

Piyathilake, C. J., Macaluso, M., Chambers, M. M., Badiga, S., Siddiqui, N. R., Bell, W. C., et al. (2014). Folate and vitamin B12 may play a critical role in lowering the HPV 16 methylation-associated risk of developing higher grades of CIN. *Cancer Prevention Research (Philadelphia, Pa.)*, 7(11), 1128–1137.

Porterfield, D. S., Dutton, G., & Gizlice, Z. (2003). Cervical cancer in North Carolina. Incidence, mortality and risk factors. *North Carolina Medical Journal*, *64*(1), 11–17.

Rainho, C. A., Kowalski, L. P., & Rogatto, S. R. (2001). Loss of imprinting and loss of heterozygosity on 11p15.5 in head and neck squamous cell carcinomas. *Head & Neck, 23*(10), 851–859.
Rainier, S., Johnson, L. A., Dobry, C. J., Ping, A. J., Grundy, P. E., & Feinberg, A. P. (1993). Relaxation of imprinted genes in human cancer. *Nature, 362*(6422), 747–749.
Ravenel, J. D., Broman, K. W., Perlman, E. J., Niemitz, E. L., Jayawardena, T. M., Bell, D. W., et al. (2001). Loss of imprinting of insulin-like growth factor-II (IGF2) gene in distinguishing specific biologic subtypes of Wilms tumor. *Journal of the National Cancer Institute, 93*(22), 1698–1703.
Reik, W., & Walter, J. (2001). Genomic imprinting: Parental influence on the genome. *Nature Reviews. Genetics, 2*, 21–32.
Rodrigues-Coutlee, C., Archambault, J., Money, D., Ramanakumar, A. V., Raboud, J., Hankins, C., et al. (2013). Human papillomavirus type 56 polymorphism in Canadian women with and without cervical lesions. *Journal of Clinical Virology, 58*(4), 660–665.
Sagasta, A., Castillo, P., Saco, A., Torne, A., Esteve, R., Marimon, L., et al. (2016). p16 staining has limited value in predicting the outcome of histological low-grade squamous intraepithelial lesions of the cervix. *Modern Pathology, 29*(1), 51–59.
Saraiya, M., Ahmed, F., Krishnan, S., Richards, T. B., Unger, E. R., & Lawson, H. W. (2007). Cervical cancer incidence in a prevaccine era in the United States, 1998-2002. *Obstetrics and Gynecology, 109*(2 Pt. 1), 360–370.
Schiff, M., Becker, T. M., Masuk, M., van Asselt-King, L., Wheeler, C. M., Altobelli, K. K., et al. (2000). Risk factors for cervical intraepithelial neoplasia in southwestern American Indian women. *American Journal of Epidemiology, 152*(8), 716–726.
Schiffman, M., & Adrianza, M. E. (2000). ASCUS-LSIL Triage Study. Design, methods and characteristics of trial participants. *Acta Cytologica, 44*(5), 726–742.
Schiffman, M. H., Bauer, H. M., Hoover, R. N., Glass, A. G., Cadell, D. M., Rush, B. B., et al. (1993). Epidemiologic evidence showing that human papillomavirus infection causes most cervical intraepithelial neoplasia. *Journal of the National Cancer Institute, 85*(12), 958–964.
Schiffman, M., & Solomon, D. (2003). Findings to date from the ASCUS-LSIL Triage Study (ALTS). *Archives of Pathology & Laboratory Medicine, 127*(8), 946–949.
Schneider, A. (1993). Pathogenesis of genital HPV infection. *Genitourinary Medicine, 69*(3), 165–173.
Sichero, L., Ferreira, S., Trottier, H., Duarte-Franco, E., Ferenczy, A., Franco, E. L., et al. (2007). High grade cervical lesions are caused preferentially by non-European variants of HPVs 16 and 18. *International Journal of Cancer, 120*(8), 1763–1768.
Sichero, L., Franco, E. L., & Villa, L. L. (2005). Different P105 promoter activities among natural variants of human papillomavirus type 18. *The Journal of Infectious Diseases, 191*(5), 739–742.
Sigurdsson, K. (1999). The Icelandic and Nordic cervical screening programs: Trends in incidence and mortality rates through 1995. *Acta Obstetricia et Gynecologica Scandinavica, 78*(6), 478–485.
Smith, J. S. (2008). Ethnic disparities in cervical cancer illness burden and subsequent care: A prospective view in managed care. *The American Journal of Managed Care, 14*(6 Suppl. 1), S193–S199.
Smith, J. S., Green, J., Berrington de Gonzalez, A., Appleby, P., Peto, J., Plummer, M., et al. (2003). Cervical cancer and use of hormonal contraceptives: A systematic review. *Lancet, 361*(9364), 1159–1167.
Smith, E. M., Johnson, S. R., Jiang, M. S., & Zaleski, S. (1991). The association between pregnancy and human papillomavirus prevalence. *Cancer Detection and Prevention, 15*(5), 397–402.

Smith, J. S., Lindsay, L., Hoots, B., Keys, J., Franceschi, S., Winer, R., et al. (2007). Human papillomavirus type distribution in invasive cervical cancer and high-grade cervical lesions: A meta-analysis update. *International Journal of Cancer, 121*(3), 621–632.

Stanczuk, G. A., Sibanda, E. N., Perrey, C., Chirara, M., Pravica, V., Hutchinson, I. V., et al. (2001). Cancer of the uterine cervix may be significantly associated with a gene polymorphism coding for increased IL-10 production. *International Journal of Cancer, 94*(6), 792–794.

Sullivan, M. J., Taniguchi, T., Jhee, A., Kerr, N., & Reeve, A. E. (1999). Relaxation of IGF2 imprinting in Wilms tumours associated with specific changes in IGF2 methylation. *Oncogene, 18*(52), 7527–7534.

Syrjanen, K., Shabalova, I., Petrovichev, N., Kozachenko, V., Zakharova, T., Pajanidi, J., et al. (2007). Smoking is an independent risk factor for oncogenic human papillomavirus (HPV) infections but not for high-grade CIN. *European Journal of Epidemiology, 22*(10), 723–735.

Szarewski, A., Jarvis, M. J., Sasieni, P., Anderson, M., Edwards, R., Steele, S. J., et al. (1996). Effect of smoking cessation on cervical lesion size. *Lancet, 347*(9006), 941–943.

Thiry, L., Vokaer, R., Detremmerie, O., De Schepper, N., Herzog, A., & Bollen, A. (1993). Cancer of the cervix, papillomavirus, contraception and tobacco. *Journal de Gynécologie, Obstétrique et Biologie de la Reproduction, 22*(5), 477–486.

Thomas, D. B., & Ray, R. M. (1995). Depot-medroxyprogesterone acetate (DMPA) and risk of invasive adenocarcinomas and adenosquamous carcinomas of the uterine cervix. WHO Collaborative Study of Neoplasia and Steroid Contraceptives. *Contraception, 52*(5), 307–312.

Torre, L. A., Siegel, R. L., Ward, E. M., & Jemal, A. (2016). Global cancer incidence and mortality rates and trends—An update. *Cancer Epidemiology, Biomarkers & Prevention, 25*(1), 16–27.

Trimble, C. L., Genkinger, J. M., Burke, A. E., Hoffman, S. C., Helzlsouer, K. J., Diener-West, M., et al. (2005). Active and passive cigarette smoking and the risk of cervical neoplasia. *Obstetrics and Gynecology, 105*(1), 174–181.

University of Zimbabwe/JHPIEGO Cervical Cancer Project. (1999). Visual inspection with acetic acid for cervical-cancer screening: Test qualities in a primary-care setting. *Lancet, 353*(9156), 869–873.

Uyeno, S., Aoki, Y., Nata, M., Sagisaka, K., Kayama, T., Yoshimoto, T., et al. (1996). IGF2 but not H19 shows loss of imprinting in human glioma. *Cancer Research, 56*(23), 5356–5359.

van den Brule, A. J., Snijders, P. J., Raaphorst, P. M., Schrijnemakers, H. F., Delius, H., Gissmann, L., et al. (1992). General primer polymerase chain reaction in combination with sequence analysis for identification of potentially novel human papillomavirus genotypes in cervical lesions. *Journal of Clinical Microbiology, 30*(7), 1716–1721.

van Roozendaal, C. E., Gillis, A. J., Klijn, J. G., van Ooijen, B., Claassen, C. J., Eggermont, A. M., et al. (1998). Loss of imprinting of IGF2 and not H19 in breast cancer, adjacent normal tissue and derived fibroblast cultures. *FEBS Letters, 437*(1–2), 107–111.

Vanakankovit, N., & Taneepanichskul, S. (2008). Effect of oral contraceptives on risk of cervical cancer. *Journal of the Medical Association of Thailand = Chotmaihet thangphaet, 91*(1), 7–12.

Varrault, A., Gueydan, C., Delalbre, A., Bellmann, A., Houssami, S., Aknin, C., et al. (2006). Zac1 regulates an imprinted gene network critically involved in the control of embryonic growth. *Developmental Cell, 11*(5), 711–722.

Verma, M. (2003). Viral genes and methylation. *Annals of the New York Academy of Sciences, 983*, 170–180.

Vidal, A. C., Henry, N. M., Murphy, S. K., Oneko, O., Nye, M., Bartlett, J. A., et al. (2014). PEG1/MEST and IGF2 DNA methylation in CIN and in cervical cancer. *Clinical & Translational Oncology*, *16*(3), 266–272.

Vidal, A. C., Murphy, S. K., Hernandez, B. Y., Vasquez, B., Bartlett, J. A., Oneko, O., et al. (2011). Distribution of HPV genotypes in cervical intraepithelial lesions and cervical cancer in Tanzanian women. *Infectious Agents and Cancer*, *6*(1), 20.

Vidal, A. C., Smith, J. S., Valea, F., Bentley, R., Gradison, M., Yarnall, K. S., et al. (2014). HPV genotypes and cervical intraepithelial neoplasia in a multiethnic cohort in the southeastern USA. *Cancer Causes & Control*, *25*(8), 1055–1062.

Villa, L. L., Sichero, L., Rahal, P., Caballero, O., Ferenczy, A., Rohan, T., et al. (2000). Molecular variants of human papillomavirus types 16 and 18 preferentially associated with cervical neoplasia. *The Journal of General Virology*, *81*(Pt. 12), 2959–2968.

Vu, T. H., Jirtle, R. L., & Hoffman, A. R. (2006). Cross-species clues of an epigenetic imprinting regulatory code for the IGF2R gene. *Cytogenetic and Genome Research*, *113*(1–4), 202–208.

Vu, T. H., Li, T., & Hoffman, A. R. (2004). Promoter-restricted histone code, not the differentially methylated DNA regions or antisense transcripts, marks the imprinting status of IGF2R in human and mouse. *Human Molecular Genetics*, *13*(19), 2233–2245.

Wallboomers, J. M., Jacobs, M. V., Manos, M. M., Bosch, F. X., Kummer, J. A., Shah, K. V., et al. (1999). Human papillomavirus is a necessary cause of invasive cancer worldwide. *The Journal of Pathology*, *189*, 12–19.

Waterland, R. A., Dolinoy, D. C., Lin, J. R., Smith, C. A., Shi, X., & Tahiliani, K. G. (2006). Maternal methyl supplements increase offspring DNA methylation at Axin fused. *Genesis*, *44*(9), 401–406.

Waterland, R. A., & Jirtle, R. L. (2003). Transposable elements: Targets for early nutritional effects on epigenetic gene regulation. *Molecular and Cellular Biology*, *23*(15), 5293–5300.

Wentzensen, N., Sherman, M. E., Schiffman, M., & Wang, S. S. (2009). Utility of methylation markers in cervical cancer early detection: Appraisal of the state-of-the-science. *Gynecologic Oncology*, *112*(2), 293–299.

Wilson, A. S., Power, B. E., & Molloy, P. L. (2007). DNA hypomethylation and human diseases. *Biochimica et Biophysica Acta*, *1775*(1), 138–162.

Winkelstein, W., Jr. (1977). Smoking and cancer of the uterine cervix: Hypothesis. *American Journal of Epidemiology*, *106*(4), 257–259.

Wisman, G. B., Nijhuis, E. R., Hoque, M. O., Reesink-Peters, N., Koning, A. J., Volders, H. H., et al. (2006). Assessment of gene promoter hypermethylation for detection of cervical neoplasia. *International Journal of Cancer*, *119*(8), 1908–1914.

Woodson, K., Flood, A., Green, L., Tangrea, J. A., Hanson, J., Cash, B., et al. (2004). Loss of insulin-like growth factor-II imprinting and the presence of screen-detected colorectal adenomas in women. *Journal of the National Cancer Institute*, *96*(5), 407–410.

Wordlaw-Stinson, L., Jones, S., Little, S., Fish, L., Vidal, A., Smith, J. S., et al. (2014). Challenges and recommendations to recruiting women who do not adhere to follow-up gynecological care. *Open Journal of Preventive Medicine*, *4*(3), 123–128.

Wu, J., Qin, Y., Li, B., He, W. Z., & Sun, Z. L. (2008). Hypomethylated and hypermethylated profiles of H19DMR are associated with the aberrant imprinting of IGF2 and H19 in human hepatocellular carcinoma. *Genomics*, *91*(5), 443–450.

Wu, M. S., Wang, H. P., Lin, C. C., Sheu, J. C., Shun, C. T., Lee, W. J., et al. (1997). Loss of imprinting and overexpression of IGF2 gene in gastric adenocarcinoma. *Cancer Letters*, *120*(1), 9–14.

Wu, H. K., Weksberg, R., Minden, M. D., & Squire, J. A. (1997). Loss of imprinting of human insulin-like growth factor II gene, IGF2, in acute myeloid leukemia. *Biochemical and Biophysical Research Communications*, *231*(2), 466–472.

Wylie, A. A., Murphy, S. K., Orton, T. C., & Jirtle, R. L. (2000). Novel imprinted DLK1/GTL2 domain on human chromosome 14 contains motifs that mimic those implicated in IGF2/H19 regulation. *Genome Research, 10*(11), 1711–1718.

Xi, L. F., Kiviat, N. B., Hildesheim, A., Galloway, D. A., Wheeler, C. M., Ho, J., et al. (2006). Human papillomavirus type 16 and 18 variants: Race-related distribution and persistence. *Journal of the National Cancer Institute, 98*(15), 1045–1052.

Xi, L. F., Koutsky, L. A., Hildesheim, A., Galloway, D. A., Wheeler, C. M., Winer, R. L., et al. (2007). Risk for high-grade cervical intraepithelial neoplasia associated with variants of human papillomavirus types 16 and 18. *Cancer Epidemiology, Biomarkers & Prevention, 16*(1), 4–10.

Xi, L. F., Schiffman, M., Koutsky, L. A., He, Z., Winer, R. L., Hulbert, A., et al. (2013). Persistence of newly detected human papillomavirus type 31 infection, stratified by variant lineage. *International Journal of Cancer, 132*(3), 549–555.

Xin, Z., Allis, C. D., & Wagstaff, J. (2001). Parent-specific complementary patterns of histone H3 lysine 9 and H3 lysine 4 methylation at the Prader-Willi syndrome imprinting center. *American Journal of Human Genetics, 69*(6), 1389–1394.

Yang, Y., Li, T., Vu, T. H., Ulaner, G. A., Hu, J. F., & Hoffman, A. R. (2003). The histone code regulating expression of the imprinted mouse Igf2r gene. *Endocrinology, 144*(12), 5658–5670.

Yu, Y., Fujii, S., Yuan, J., Luo, R. Z., Wang, L., Bao, J., et al. (2003). Epigenetic regulation of ARHI in breast and ovarian cancer cells. *Annals of the New York Academy of Sciences, 983*, 268–277.

Yu, Y., Xu, F., Peng, H., Fang, X., Zhao, S., Li, Y., et al. (1999). NOEY2 (ARHI), an imprinted putative tumor suppressor gene in ovarian and breast carcinomas. *Proceedings of the National Academy of Sciences of the United States of America, 96*(1), 214–219.

Yuan, J., Luo, R. Z., Fujii, S., Wang, L., Hu, W., Andreeff, M., et al. (2003). Aberrant methylation and silencing of ARHI, an imprinted tumor suppressor gene in which the function is lost in breast cancers. *Cancer Research, 63*(14), 4174–4180.

Zhao, Z., Tavoosidana, G., Sjolinder, M., Gondor, A., Mariano, P., Wang, S., et al. (2006). Circular chromosome conformation capture (4C) uncovers extensive networks of epigenetically regulated intra- and interchromosomal interactions. *Nature Genetics, 38*(11), 1341–1347.

# INDEX

Note: Page numbers followed by "*f*" indicate figures, and "*t*" indicate tables.

## T



## W

FSC
www.fsc.org
MIX
Papier | Fördert gute Waldnutzung
FSC® C083411

Kolibri 360 GmbH
Ferdinand-Jühlke-Straße 7
99095 Erfurt, Deutschland
produktsicherheit@kolibri360.de